ADVANCE PRAISE FOR

Curriculum Studies in the Age of Covid-19: Stories of the Unbearable

"As a hospital chaplain in the era of Covid-19, Dr. Marla Morris provides care to the souls of patients, paying tribute to their untold stories inevitably marked by inexplicable suffering and sadness. Because such stories cannot be captured in the sterile language of the clinical chart, she turns to such writers as Terry Tempest Williams, John Gunther, and Louise DeSalvo to gain insights into the profound and contradictory experiences of illness she witnesses. But Dr. Morris is not only a chaplain. She is also a curriculum theorist who enacts *currere*, a way of viewing the world of Covid in deeply personal ways through her relationships with patients, their families, and their caregivers; and in larger sociopolitical, theological, and spiritual spheres. And there's more: she is also a philosopher who turns to the theoretical frameworks of Derrida, Camus, and Serres among others to explore how their relevance illuminates the pandemic in ways not examined before.

Curriculum Studies in the Age of Covid-19: Stories of the Unbearable is brilliant, far-reaching scholarship marked by the sensitivity and passion of Dr. Morris, a work that ultimately helps us all honor what she calls in these pages 'the unbearable stories' of Covid-19."
—Delese Wear, PhD, Professor Emerita, Department of Family and Community Medicine, Northeast Ohio Medical University

"Marla Morris has written a book that is a gift for all of us who live at the intersection of medicine, philosophy, literature, and being human. Drawing on an astonishing range of scholarship and an equally astonishing range of lived experience in the middle of the COVID pandemic, Dr. Morris manages to enliven the too-often abstract world of academic reflection on illness and death with clear-eyed witness to the agony at the heart of this crisis. In the evolution of her arguments about unbearable stories, she brings a sophisticated structure for interpretation of these stories in the often-chaotic realm of plague medicine. She does this with the wisdom of an experienced educator, the grace of an experienced chaplain, and the skilled eye of an experienced storyteller. I worked with her in the trenches of a hospital serving thirty-six southern rural counties during the worst of the COVID pandemic. I was grateful for her work as a chaplain in the rooms of our patients and I am ever-grateful to her as a philosopher who has given us a profound way of drilling down on complex lived experiences in this difficult season."
—Raymond Barfield, MD, PhD, Palliative Care Physician, Memorial University Medical Center, Savannah, Georgia; Mercer Medical School, Savannah and Macon, Georgia

Curriculum Studies in the Age of Covid-19

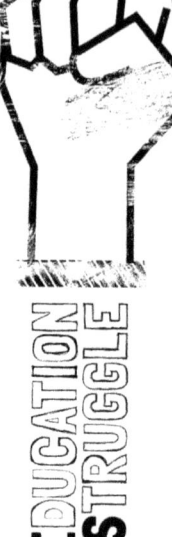

Narrative, Dialogue, and the Political Production of Meaning

Michael A. Peters & Peter McLaren
Series Editors

Vol. 24

The Education and Struggle series is part of the Peter Lang Education list.
Every volume is peer reviewed and meets
the highest quality standards for content and production.

PETER LANG
New York • Bern • Berlin
Brussels • Vienna • Oxford • Warsaw

Marla Morris

Curriculum Studies in the Age of Covid-19

Stories of the Unbearable

PETER LANG
New York • Bern • Berlin
Brussels • Vienna • Oxford • Warsaw

Library of Congress Cataloging-in-Publication Control Number: 2022016518

Bibliographic information published by **Die Deutsche Nationalbibliothek.**
Die Deutsche Nationalbibliothek lists this publication in the "Deutsche
Nationalbibliografie"; detailed bibliographic data are available
on the Internet at http://dnb.d-nb.de/.

ISSN 2168-6432 (print)
ISSN 2168-6459 (online)
ISBN 978-1-4331-9746-8 (hardcover)
ISBN 978-1-4331-9698-0 (paperback)
ISBN 978-1-4331-9744-4 (ebook pdf)
ISBN 978-1-4331-9745-1 (epub)
DOI 10.3726/b19735

© 2022 Peter Lang Publishing, Inc., New York
80 Broad Street, 5th floor, New York, NY 10004
www.peterlang.com

All rights reserved.
Reprint or reproduction, even partially, in all forms such as microfilm,
xerography, microfiche, microcard, and offset strictly prohibited.

Dedication

This book is dedicated to William F. Pinar. Bill is my dear friend, mentor and PhD advisor. In 1999 I graduated from Louisiana State University with PhD in hand under Bill's tutelage. Today I am entering my 22nd year as a professor at Georgia Southern University. Even though much time has passed since those amazing days at LSU, the memories of studying with Bill are etched in my heart still. Bill has continually inspired me throughout *The Stages on Life's Way*—as Kierkegaard would put it. This book is written with gratitude to Bill beyond what language can capture.

Contents

Introduction: Metaphors of the Desert: A Curriculum of Crisis   1

1   Clinical Narratives and Stultification   29

2   Speculative Fabulation and Unbearable Stories   47

3   Jacques Derrida's Concepts: Metaphors for Unbearable Stories   65

4   Thomas Merton's Crisis of The Unspeakable   89

5   The Unbearable Stories of Terry Tempest Williams, Joan Didion and Derrick Jensen   111

6   The Unbearable Stories of Anton Boisen, Louise DeSalvo and John Gunther   139

7   Albert Camus' Relevance for Unbearable Stories of the Covid Pandemic   161

8   Michel Serres' Relevance for Unbearable Stories of the Covid
    Pandemic   187

    References   207
    Index   217

Introduction: Metaphors of the Desert: A Curriculum of Crisis

Palm Springs is situated in the middle of a vast orange desert. It is as if one is walking into the Sahara. But this is not the Sahara. The Sahara is in Africa. Palm Springs is in California. This is the desert in Palm Springs, California. Nearby, The Joshua Tree National Park winds around and around a ghostly, forbidding moonlike landscape—or moonscape. There is something strange about this place. On a National Government Park website The Joshua Tree description reads: "Two distinct desert ecosystems, the Mojave and the Colorado, come together in Joshua Tree National Park…. a land sculpted by strong winds and occasional torrents of rain…. [with] surreal geological features" (nps.gov, May 22, 2019 author unknown). Surreal, indeed. What comes to mind as well is the rock band U2 whose album called *The Joshua Tree* influenced many musicians of my generation. Valentina Magli (March 6, 2017), who connects U2's album to the spiritual aspect of the Joshua Tree in Palm Springs remarks: "The [Joshua Tree] was named by early Mormon Settlers, after the Old Testament [sic, Hebrew Scriptures] prophet Joshua, as its branches reminded them of Joshua raising his arms to pray" (Hotpress.com, March 6, 2017). From Palm Springs to the Joshua Tree National Park—reminiscent of a Sci-Fi film—postmodern windmills dot a moonlike backdrop.

My partner Mary Doll and I joined my PhD advisor—William F. Pinar with his partner Jeff Turner—in Palm Springs for a New Year's Celebration. This was a vacation that was supposed to be joyous. And it was. Yet, in waves, I was hit by grief. I began walking through Palm Springs by myself when memories of horrible things—seemingly out of nowhere—struck me while reminiscing about San Diego. I lived in San Diego from 1978 to 1980. Those were my last two years of high school. Grief overtook me. Out of nowhere I became overwhelmed by the memories of the death of a friend from Escondido and the more recent the death of my mother. I broke down looking up at the Palm Trees against the orange sky of the desert, unbeknownst to anyone. A long rush of ancient unfelt emotions hit me like a boulder.

Thomas Merton (1981) writes: "mysticism is born of a theological crisis" (p. 107).

Although this was not a mystical or theological crisis, breaking down in the middle of the street was an existential crisis.

Thomas Merton's (1981) words—and my existential crisis—began the long journey of writing this book. For me, the urgency of writing is akin to crisis; this book was "born" in crisis. A crisis is always already ecological as it is an attempt to heal what is long broken. Compounded grief—coping with the loss of a friend and my mother—had arrived at a very strange time, belatedly. Perhaps it arrived too late. There are deaths that do not heal over. Memories of death(s)—from years past—get buried in the ashes of repression. The strange moonscape backdrop of Palm Springs and visiting the Joshua Tree National Park brought unrelenting grief.

I was stunned at my own crushed psyche while walking through Palm Springs. Perhaps there is a relation between walking, thinking and repressed memory rising. Grief welled up out of nowhere. Clock-Time, as I call it, does not exist in the flow that is memory.

It seems odd that it was the landscape that evoked distant and painful memories; memories of death emerge when they want to—not when one is ready, psychologically, to remember. That desert landscape—forbidding and barren—became the place where I had to face what I could not. Against the backdrop of that Sahara-like sky, Terry Tempest Williams' (2001) words came to mind: "I am desert. I am mountains. I am Great Salt Lake. There are other languages spoken by the wind, water, and wings" (p. 29). Although the Great Salt Lake and Palm Springs are vastly different, Terry Tempest Williams' words spoke to me. It is not insignificant that Williams grew up in a Mormon family. Mormons initially named that place in Palm Springs (where I found myself in psychic disarray) The Joshua Tree. Williams' words resonate with the landscape of the desert.

It is not lost on me that all the women in Williams' family died of cancer. It is not lost on me that Williams' mother died of ovarian cancer. I almost died of ovarian cancer in 2016. When the surgeon sat down next to my hospital bed and said the words ovarian cancer, I forgot that I had ever read Terry Tempest Williams. I had no idea what ovarian cancer meant, even though I taught Williams' (2001) *Refuge* many times. All I heard was the word cancer. I heard nothing else. Everything went blank.

Currere—the Latin root of curriculum—is key to William F. Pinar's reconceptualization of curriculum studies, a paradigm shift in the history of curriculum as a field. *Currere* suggests looking within but it also points to the socio-political. *Currere* is about one's relationship to oneself, to others, to the land, to the larger ecosphere. For me, *currere* is a deeply ecological concept. For me, *currere* is also a deeply theological concept. *Currere*—as a concept—is not incompatible with the theological, or the spiritual.

Currere as a lived concept was enacted, for me, as a deeply eco-theological crisis in the face of memory and death. *Currere*—for Pinar—has relations to Edmund Husserl's notion of *lebenswelt* –or lived experience. The life-world is also about death. *Currere*, thereby is not only one's relation to lived experience, but it is also one's relationship to death, especially one's *aversion* to death. *Currere* is about one's relationship to the divine as well as one's *aversion* to the divine. *Currere* is related to that which is numinous, to that which is holy, as Rudolph Otto (1958) put it. The holy—as numinous—is not light; the holy means holy terror.

Many who have suffered the horrors of cancer say: There *was* the time before cancer; there *is* the time after cancer. After a cancer diagnosis, everything that came before is somehow blurred, lost, or repressed. Cancer is the shadow of the object. Perhaps it was the cancer diagnosis in 2016 that put on hold—for me—the mourning of my friend and my mother. A part of me died in 2016 when the bad news was delivered. Part of my memory just fell off of a cliff. But memory has a way of catching up with you. My "theological crisis" (Merton, 1981, p. 107)—the return of the repressed—compounded the holy terror of death.

This book is an attempt to hammer out—as Nietzsche (2008) might put it—complicated grief as a "theological crisis" (Merton, 1981, p. 107)—not just my own theological crisis or my own story of dealing with death, but the stories of others and how they cope or do not cope with death.

As I began writing the book, the covid-19 pandemic had not yet arrived. It was, as Derrida would put it, to come. Thus the book grew into a testimony to those who lost their lives during the pandemic. What began as an autobiography grew into a biography of sorts. What began as a virus elsewhere became a virus everywhere. This horror and tragedy was not inevitable and did not have to get played out in the tragic way that it did. Nothing is pre-determined; things could have happened otherwise.

This book is an archive of the present and the past; this book is about what I call stories of the unbearable. Because there is little precedent for the stories of those lost to covid, it is difficult to know how to navigate through this tragedy. I am not a historian, nor am I an archivist. I examine—throughout—unbearable stories in the form of biography—as I interweave my own autobiography—with memoirs of those who have suffered horrors that are not unrelated to covid but that are not directly about covid. One must begin somewhere. But the problem is, is that there is no place to begin—because this pandemic is unlike any other. Thus, I begin with unbearable stories that are tangentially related to what it is that families (who have lost loved ones to covid) are currently suffering through. This might be a problematic approach because stories of illness and death should not be compared.

So where do I begin? That is a political, philosophical, theological and curricular question. Although my approach might be problematic, I begin where I can best make connections to our current crisis, that is, covid-19. The task is to archive covid as it is unfolding in the present, because once unfolding memories are gone, history becomes stultified. Memories—of this horror—will fade over time.

The question of what history is, is also problematic. When does history begin? Is an unfolding present history? When does history become history? Does the present moment count as history? The minutes that slip by are indeed always already history. I did not want to wait until the pandemic was over to write this. I wanted to archive what I could in the now so that in the future these words will be marked by their closeness in time to this event: these words give us something to hold onto.

Although the 1918 flu epidemic has been well documented, especially in the medical literature, not many people lived long enough to tell their stories—from a first-person perspective. Perhaps medical anthropologists will make connections between the 1918 flu epidemic and the current covid crisis; but at this historical juncture it is, perhaps, still too early to tell what connections can or cannot be made.

Through the intersection of curriculum theory, politics, theology and philosophy of education, this book is an attempt to confront the real, as painful as that may be. I navigate the complexities of curriculum theory, philosophy, politics and theology as both a professor of education and as a hospital chaplain—with boots on the ground—wading through the muck that is Covid-19. Thus, I am approaching the pandemic from several different angles. Theory and praxis, here go hand-in-glove. As a university professor I have witnessed the politicization that is covid as a tragic affair; professors (and school teachers) are dying, college students are vanishing, and now school children are getting sick, some dying. The lack of accountability on the part of politicians and university administrators beholden to state politics, the lack of unions especially in the Southern part of the United States, and the lax policies on masks and vaccines in both schools and universities have resulted in the needless deaths of untold numbers of people. School teachers and university professors—who are not unionized—have little power to rise up against state institutions that do not follow or respect science. Power—is not merely a concept—it is real. The lack of power—that most professors and teachers have experienced—has become, in fact, a deadly game. Go to work and risk life. Quit and risk bankruptcy and/or the loss of a career. Marx once remarked, in response to the theoretical writings of Feuerbach the 19th-century theologian, that it is not enough to write about the world, one must change the world. But can writing about the world really change the world? Can writing about the world change some piece of the world? Only time will tell.

I am writing this with the aim of changing the world. I am writing this book because it is my duty and responsibility—as both an academic and hospital chaplain—to archive this crisis. It is the archive that matters in the end. The archive is not static; it is an ever-moving process, an endless stream of disruptions, interruptions, confusions and moments of despair. This book was written in a stream of confusion: because that is how history is lived.

In 2018, two years after my cancer diagnosis I entered a program called Clinical Pastoral Education (known as CPE) at Memorial University Medical Center Hospital in Savannah, Georgia. This chaplaincy program is under the auspices of the College of Pastoral Supervision and Psychotherapy (known as CPSP); it is rooted in psychodynamic psychoanalysis. CPSP is not primarily religious in nature. In fact, religion has very little to do with my work as a chaplain. CPSP chaplaincy is not about checklists or standardized jargon. Hospital administrators, however, prefer standardized clinical narratives. However, CPSP fights these trends. CPSP is one of the few chaplaincy programs that is in sync with my work as an academic, as a curriculum theorist. The form of chaplaincy in which

I am engaged dovetails Pinar's reconceptualization. Chaplaincy is both a theoretical and clinical field.

Curriculum studies—as Reconceptualized—has its early roots in psychoanalysis (see Pinar, 1975; Grumet, 1988) and spirituality, e.g. the works of James Macdonald (1995) and Dwayne Huebner (1999), to name but a few. Like the fights that go on in CPSP against the pressures of standardization in hospital settings, curriculum studies is *still* an ongoing battle against Ralph Tyler's (1959) paradigm—referred to as the Tyler rationale—a model of thought that standardizes outcomes and forecloses on intellectual labor.

My work as a clinical chaplain has been greatly influenced by William F. Pinar's (2009) *The worldliness of a cosmopolitan education: Passionate lives in public service*. Pinar (2009) writes: "academic study and lived experience subjectively reconstructed provide passages from private preoccupations to public service" (p. xii). It has long been a struggle to figure out how to live as an academic while also doing clinical work in the field (of the hospital). Both my life in the professoriate and my clinical life as a hospital chaplain are, at root, about doing good work; in the Jewish tradition, this is called *Tikkun*.

Being a Jewish intellectual means connecting theory with praxis; that praxis must be theoretical. The juggling act—between theory and praxis—had been a conundrum for me——until I got cancer. Cancer changed everything; it turned my life upside down. Because I got cancer and survived—I felt I owed a debt of gratitude to the very hospital—and medical team—that saved my life. Ovarian cancer is not one that many survive. But because my cancer was caught early, I have been given the gift of time. That time I will use to do what I consider to be a duty and responsibility. Unlike many, I have an insider's view on what goes on in covid wards—as a chaplain—I have witnessed covid in a way others cannot.

Living a double life as scholar and hospital chaplain, I am—as Pinar (2009) puts it—engaging in the world, living out a passionate life in public service. Like Pinar, Edward Said (2001) writes about being a scholar-in-the-world. Said (2001) states: "I didn't then (and don't now) pretend for a moment that reading and writing are in themselves otherworldly; of course they're not, but the question is how are they in the world, and how can they be in the world—a terrifyingly complex question" (p. 22). Reading and writing, chaplaincy and the professoriate are ways of Being-in-the-world. What is terrifying—is not, as Said puts it, how reading and writing can be put to use in the world—but witnessing the deaths of untold numbers from covid; being witness to the ever-going parade of body-bags being taken to the morgue.

This chapter is roughly divided into three meditations.[1] The first meditation concerns metaphors of the desert and how those metaphors evoke *thoughts* of death. The second meditation concerns what I term an ecology of death. Here, I explore what facing death means *experientially*. Of course, thought and experience cannot be separated, both are one, even if thought-as-experience is deferred and delayed, what Derrida terms *differance*. The third meditation—at the end of this introductory chapter—outlines the chapters to follow so that the reader knows what is to come, as Derrida might put it.

Metaphors of the Desert: First Meditation

Perhaps it is no accident that Paul Bowles' (1949/1977) novel about death—*The Sheltering Sky*—takes place in the Saharan desert. A blurb on the back jacket cover of the book reads: Bowles' "etches the limits of human reason and intelligence—perhaps even the limits of human life—when they touch the unfathomable and impassive cruelty of the desert" (n.p., author unknown, 1947/1977 ECCO Press Edition). Port and Kit—the two protagonists in the book—live in a cruel and heartless—but seemingly necessary but unhinged—relationship of love and hate. They explore the Saharan desert together—interrupted by a character named Tunner—who seems always in the way of the drama at hand. As a prelude to death, Bowles (1949/1977) says of Port: "The idea that at each successive moment he was deeper into the Sahara than he had been a moment before, he was leaving behind all familiar things… " (p. 109). Port was leaving the behind familiar because he was dying.

Port's cruelty toward Kit is as cruel as the desert landscape. But this twisted and cruel relation between Port and Kit seems oddly necessary. These two characters are inseparable even though—and perhaps because—they hate one another. There is a psychic desert between them as they are cold to one another and yet need one another in that coldness. And deserts like the Sahara get ghastly cold at night but are hot as hell during the day. Carlo Carretto (1964/1990)—who was a school teacher in Italy for a time—left teaching behind; he ventured out into the Sahara to live a monk-like existence in the desert. Carretto (1964/1990) comments that "It seems strange to speak of cold in the desert, but it is so; in fact the Sahara is often called 'a cold country where it is very hot in the sun'" (p. 3). Interestingly, in Bowles' novel, Port complains that he is cold—even during the day—when the temperature is very hot. Port is cold—probably—because he is ill, perhaps from meningitis: he eventually succumbs to his illness. Port dies in the desert. Kit locks the door behind her—leaving Port dead on the floor—and just walks away. Does Kit desert Port? It feels that way. But that is what people do. They walk away from the dead. What else can one do? Still, leaving a body behind seems a desertion of sorts.

Kit's inability to cope with Port's death leads her to become—willingly—a sex slave to desert peoples. Kit is thrown into a culture about which she knows nothing. When her sexual escapades turn nightmarish, she barely escapes with her life. Bowles' narrative becomes increasingly sado-masochistic. Visceral brutality –and Kit's willingness to engage in this brutality—shocks. By engaging in such brutality willingly, it seems that symbolically, Kit abandons her (self). Kit's self-abandonment mirrors the abandonment of the Other—and in this case that Other is Port.

John Chryssavgis (2008) notes that the word "desert" in Greek "literally means 'abandonment'" (p. 33). In the book of *Leviticus* "The desert signified death" (p. 33). Bowles' novel deals both with death and abandonment—as Kit locks the door behind her, leaving Port behind. Bowles intimates that—in some strange way—Kit abandoned Port too soon. A fitting end to a tragically cruel, twisted sado-masochistic relationship.

I have meditated for years on Bowles' (1949/1977) *The Sheltering Sky* because I do not understand it. However, two things strike me. One: the title. What does the sky shelter? Port says to Kit, "the sky here's very strange. I often have the sensation when I look at it that it's a solid thing up there, protecting us from what's behind" (p. 101). Kit asks Port, "But what *is* [emphasis in the original] behind" (p. 101)? Port answers: "Nothing, I suppose. Just darkness. Absolute night" (p. 101). The sky shelters us—ironically—from nothing. Absolute night is death; nothing shelters us from death. And that's where religion comes in. In one way, religion is an attempt to shelter the psyche from what it cannot bear: Death. The idea of resurrection—which is not unique to Christianity— suggests that death *is not* death. Being resurrected means going somewhere else; resurrection is a movement of transcendence. But if psyche is going somewhere else by transcending this life, is that death at all? In another way, theology—and not religion[2]—can be an attempt to confront the unthinkable. Thomas Merton's (1981) "theological crisis" is an attempt to confront the "unspeakable." Bowles' (1949/1977) *The Sheltering Sky* can be read as a theological shattering, an attempt to confront the unbearable.

The second issue Bowles' (1949/1977) raises is that there is a wedge—philosophically—between *thinking* about the death of the self and *experiencing* the death of the Other. Psyche cannot think or experience its non-existence, let alone the non-existence of the Other. After a person dies, in my work as a hospital chaplain, I have witnessed families barely able to leave the body behind. The most excruciating moment for many is leaving the hospital.

The narrator—in reference to Kit—says, "She did not remember their many conversations built around the idea of death, perhaps because no idea of death has anything in common with the presence of death.... one can *be* anything but *dead*" (p. 237). It is because "any one can be anything but dead" that philosophy begins with death, Socrates intimates; death is the philosopher's stone. But most people are not philosophers and even if they are, the lived experience of death is not the same as thinking about it philosophically.

The narratives of many religion(s) begin with origin stories. Those who study religion(s) do not usually start with stories of endings. Endings come later. Death, that is, or the eschaton, the ending, comes at the end of the narrative. (Religions are narratives, or stories; some say mythologies, even.)

The end, or the eschaton, emerges, in what is called apocalyptic literature (s), which are quite ancient, in fact. There are many apocalyptic literatures, but— strangely—there is only one book that was included in the Christian Scriptures dealing with the apocalypse. The Hebrew scriptures begin with origin stories (in the beginning there was light; Adam and Eve walking through the garden are origin stories). Some theologians suggest that (in the beginning there was light) was actually historically older than the rest of the book of Genesis. Some Biblical scholars—who work from what is called the historical-critical method, suggest that the P source, or the Priestly source (or Jewish priests) placed—and let there be light—first, even though the story is probably older than the rest of the narrative in the book of Genesis. Interestingly, some theologians argue that the story of Adam and Eve walking through the garden was probably written by women.

It is notable that the Christian scriptures end with an apocalypse.[3] These debates—about which origin story came first and why the Book of Revelation— about the apocalypse—is even in the bible to begin with—are beyond the scope of this book.[4]

The Desert as Metaphor of the Sublime

The desert is a cruel place where nuclear bombs were tested in the 1950s and resulted in countless numbers of deaths in the West from cancer (see Terry Tempest Williams (2001)). The desert is a cruel place, for those attempting to make the trek across the southern border, as Luis Alberto Urrea (2004) reports.

Untold numbers have died on the southern border; The Devil's Highway—about which Urrea (2004) writes—is littered with memories of those who died there.

Contrarily, the desert is also a place of devastating beauty, vibrant wildlife, heartbreaking vistas. The desert, therefore, is the penultimate example of the sublime. This concept—the sublime—refers to the paradoxical condition of encountering beauty and terror simultaneously. And yet, somehow these concepts—beauty and terror—do not square: the terror that is death is not beautiful.[5]

The desert, as Albert Camus (1955/1983) might put it, is a metaphor for "life without consolation" (p. 60). Camus (1955/1983) asks: "can thought live in those deserts" (p. 22)? Can life be lived without consolation? The absurd—or life lived without consolation—is, for Camus, the human condition. Facing death means facing it without gloss, without cliches, without consolation. Nothing can console a mother who lost her child to covid. In fact, to suggest that there are consoling words to offer is irresponsible and unconscionable. The worst thing a chaplain can do is to utter false consolations, or false hope, or utter trite expressions when there is nothing one can say; there is nothing to say. The unsaid is better left unsaid. Death has its own language; chaplains must allow the silent non-language of devastation to speak.

Against Nihilism: The Desert as Mirror

It is reported that weary desert travelers see mirages, or hallucinations. This is perhaps due to heat exhaustion. Mirages are mirrors. They are mirrors or wish-fantasies, as Freud might put it. One wishes for water; one sees water. Yet, no water exists. Mirages are mirrors of fear. What one fears one sees; whether what is seen is real or not. If one fears snakes, one sees them whether they are real or not. The mind is a mirror; the desert mirage is a mirror-of-the-mind. But the psyche is not glass; it is anything but clear.[5] The mirror-of-the-mind is murky.

Theologian Karl Barth famously asked the question: What am I to do? Thomas Merton asked: What am I living for? Camus asked: what is the point of Sisyphus' struggle? On her deathbed, it is reported that Gertrude Stein asked: What is the question? Deeply curricular, theological and philosophical questions directly connect to what the desert of death asks of us.

Camus (1956/1991), in *The Rebel*, states: "Metaphysical rebellion is a claim, motivated by the concept of a complete unity, against the suffering of life and death and a protest against the human condition for its incompleteness, thanks to death… " (p. 24). The "incompleteness" and suffering that is endured, however, does not justify nihilism—Camus contends.

Metaphors of the Desert Theology

Camus and Bowles both wrote fiction. Camus was also a journalist and a philosopher. The desert as a metaphor was important to both of these writers. Fiction and philosophy (together) might open avenues for thinking through the desert as a theological metaphor. Theologians, in fact, have historically taken the desert as a central metaphor. In fact, Thomas Merton (1960)—perhaps the most renowned Trappist Monk of the 20th century—introduced lay people to the literature (s) of the Desert Fathers of the 4th century CE.

Merton (1960) writes: "when the "world" became officially Christian" (p. 4)—when Constantine the Emperor of Rome converted to Christianity declaring it the "official" State religion—those who fled to the desert became troubled by the real possibility of Christian nation-building. Rome—under Constantine—became a Christian state. To Christianize a state seemed—at least to the desert fathers—antithetical to Christian life.

Christology and Orthodoxy

Christology—or the study—and codification—of who Jesus was—led to the banishment of what the Christian State of Rome considered to be heretics. The Nicaean Creed (325 CE) served to codify orthodoxy and attempted to rid Rome of heretics.

The Greek term *Homoousious*—as part of the Nicaean Creed—codified who and what Jesus was in relation to God. *Homoousious* is a concept that suggests that Jesus was one (*homo*) in substance (*ousious*) with God. Contrarily, the heterodox position—one that the heretic Arius touted—created political divisions among early Christians that the Church Fathers feared. Arius—who held a dissenting position on the meaning of *homoousious*—claimed that Jesus was not the same substance as God; rather Jesus was a "creature" (Harmless, 2004, p. 95) and "there was a time when he was not" (Harmless, 2004, p. 95). What this suggests is that Jesus was merely human, a creature, like all other human beings. If there was a time "when he was not" Jesus was born into the world. But before his birth, Jesus did not exist; therefore Jesus—as Arius argued—was not eternal.

Arius asked: How could a human being be the same in substance (*homoousious*) with God, if God is eternal? Jesus suffered and died—in the flesh—on the cross as a human being. God, if he is eternal, does not die on a cross; therefore, Jesus could not be one and the same with God. Arius implied, therefore, that Jesus was human—not divine—. This was basically a Jewish position. Although there were some early Christians who called themselves Jewish Christians; eventually they were deemed heretical.

The purpose of The Council of Nicaea was an attempt to put the Arian controversy to bed, to rid the Christian state of heretics. However, the Council of Nicaea only led to schisms: more controversies were to follow. The trinitarian controversy created even more schisms.

Thomas Merton (1960)—over time—changed his position on why the desert fathers fled when Rome became a Christian state. Jon M. Sweeney (2019) points out that Merton argued (when he changed his position on this issue) the following: "The idea that vocations to the desert came with the Edict of Constantine [313 CE] is not quite accurate. There were already many hermits in the desert before that. St. Antony embraced the hermit life [in] about 270, and went into the desert at Pispar [in]about 285. He had gathered many disciples around him before 313" (cited in Sweeney, 2019, p. 24). So if the desert fathers fled—before 313 CE when Rome became a Christian State under Constantine—what inspired them to venture into the desert in the first place?

William Harmless (2004) notes that The desert fathers, most famously Antony—whose story was told by Athanasius (1980)—wanted nothing to do with becoming "clergy." Harmless (2004) points out that—"Antony and his disciples were not clergy. In fact, monks resisted becoming clergy…. the monastic movement [was] a potentially churchless Christianity" (pp. 93-94). Antony seemed a free spirit. His wandering into the desert was perhaps an event that imitated Christ's self-actualization in the desert while tempted by demons. Jesus the Christ—as he was called—won out over temptations, as the story is told. Many thought that his overcoming temptations proved that he was, in fact, the son of God. However—at the time—there were many who called themselves son(s) of God. This was a common phrase. But for some reason, Jesus who became *the Christ*—signifying his divinity—captured culture in a way that is almost inexplicable. Entire cultures changed because of the story, the myth, the legend of Jesus—the man who wandered into the desert.

It is no accident that in the history of Christian theology, a debate raged for decades over what is called the quest for the historical Jesus. Some suggest that theologians became obsessed with proving that Jesus was the Christ because perhaps they doubted—secretly—that this person (Jesus) existed at all. Of course, this claim is still considered heretical. Doubt and anxiety perhaps drove this debate. Before Jesus became the Christ (meaning the divine one), he was called Rabbi Joshua. This name—Joshua—is not insignificant especially for Mormons who settled in the Western United States. Mormons, recall, named the tree outside of Palm Springs—which looks as if it were in prayer—the Joshua Tree. The Joshua National Park was designated as a national landmark by President Teddy Roosevelt's conservation initiatives. Sadly, in 2019, according to Liam Stack—writer for the *New York Times*—the Joshua tree(s) were destroyed (there were actually several trees designated as Joshua trees) by looters during a government shutdown. Park Rangers, according to Stack, say that it might take "centuries to regrow" the trees (Stack, NY Times, January 29, 2019, nytimes.com).

The desert has long symbolized, for Christians and perhaps other religious traditions, a place of self-actualization; a place of trial and testimony of faith. Antony—became legendary as one of the earliest monks who roamed the desert imitating Christ. Robert Ellsberg (2018) writes that Thomas Merton resonated with the desert fathers—like Antony—. For Merton—according to Ellsberg (2018)—the desert fathers (like Antony) represented heterodoxy. Merton intimates that "What the [desert] Fathers sought most of all was their own true self, in Christ. And in order to do this, they had to reject completely the false, formal self, fabricated under social compulsion in the 'world'. They sought a way to God that was uncharted and freely chosen, not inherited from others who had mapped it out beforehand" (Merton, cited in Ellsberg, 2018, p. 39).

The fragmented texts scholars have access to today do bear this out. However, Gregory of Nazianzus argued that Athanasius' Antony actually introduced "rule[s]" for how to be a monk; the legend of Antony was actually the beginning of the story of the "rule of monastic life" (Harmless, 2004, p. 69). But that is not how the story of Antony reads at all. If anything, Antony's story is shot through with fantasy and even perhaps hallucinations. Tall tales of dragons walking on crocodiles, visions of monsters, Antony's miraculous survival in a tomb—and other strange stories—hardly read like "rules on how to be a monk" or a how-to manual on how to be a monk. Antony's writings could be considered an early form of magical realism, in fact, or fable.

The Rule of St. Benedict—(a book of daily regiments, rules and routines that Benedictine monks follow to this day) might have emerged out of the Catholic church's desire to control monks so that they might not stray into heretical territory. The Rule of St. Benedict reads like a military manual. On Monday monks read this, on Tuesday monks read that, on Wednesday monks read this and so on.

In the morning monks say prayers, attend to chores, eat together, do more chores, pray at designated times during the day, eat dinner together, pray and retire at a sanctioned hour each evening. Monastic life is much like military life. The monastic life—at least for some of the orders, like the Benedictines—is about discipline, regimentation and structure. There are exceptions to this, though.

Today, some Benedictines teach in universities, live in cities outside the walls of the monastery, compete in piano competitions, and perform with symphony orchestras. Thomas Merton, though, belonged to the Cistercian Order; he was a Trappist Monk—not a Benedictine—which is perhaps the most severe sect of monastic life, for the Trappists do not speak.

However, Merton's superiors encouraged him to write, publish and travel, despite that silence is a very important vow that Trappist Monks take. Merton was tormented by his double life, his need to live a life in silent meditation, and his need to write. Merton doubted —at every step on the way—his decision to become a Trappist Monk. It was his doubt and anxiety, his struggles with his vocation, with which readers identified. Merton presented himself as a vulnerable man. It was his vulnerability—perhaps—that attracted so many readers. Merton's (1998) autobiography, *The Seven Storey Mountain*, was read worldwide; in fact, 100,000 copies were sold soon after the book was published in the late 1940s. Some consider Merton's autobiography a modern-day classic akin to Augustine's (1961) *Confessions*. Merton was not only deeply religious he was also deeply political and outspoken against the Vietnam War. Merton's politics and religious calling, his doubts and frustrations, his activism and asceticism still draw in readers to this day. His is a fascinating study of a conflicted and contradictory life. The way in which he lived inside of this conflict, inside of his own contradictory aspirations, fascinates. Merton followed that path of Antony the free spirit who wandered into the desert. Merton was a free spirit, indeed, even as he was bound by his calling as a Trappist monk.

Along with Athanasius' Antony, Benedicta Ward (1975) points out that John Cassian—who lived around 360-445 CE—wrote about the desert fathers. *The Sayings of the Desert Fathers and Mothers, or Apophthegmata Patrium* (which is a compilation of writings by many persons living in the desert in around the 4th century CE)—according to Harmless (2004)—contain "borrowings" (p. 71) from Hebrew and Christian Scripture and from philosophers. Interestingly scholars claim that Antony's tall tales might have been borrowed from other literatures. Harmless (2004) points out that "Richard Reitzenstein and other classics scholars found a spate of parallels and borrowings... [most interestingly from] Lucian's quirky holy man, Pancretes [who] spent years underground in the tombs of Egypt, studying occult sciences under Isis, and then emerged from his mystic initiation to demonstrate his powers by riding around on crocodiles" (p. 71). Like Pancrete, Antony lived in a tomb and rode on the backs of crocodiles—so the stories go.

Importantly, Athanasius's book on Antony ends this way: "Neither from writings, nor from pagan wisdom, nor from some craft was Antony acclaimed, but on account of religion alone. That this was something given by God that no one would deny" (p. 98). However, Antony does lean on pagan wisdom, (witch) craft and magic. Antony—according to Athanasius—fought "dragon[s]" (p. 34) and fought "demons" which "were changed into forms of beasts and reptiles [such as]... the appearances of lions, bears, leopards, bulls, and serpents, asps, scorpions and wolves" (p. 38). The "demons" "creat[ed] apparitions" (p. 41). "Mobs" and "phantasms" "work their fraud by being transfigured" (p. 53). It is clear—nonetheless—that Athanasius made a point of stating—in no uncertain terms—that Antony did not, in fact, engage in witchcraft or magic. But one might wonder why Athanasius felt the need to state this at all. Athanasius—perhaps—wanted to protect the legend of Antony so that the church would not dismiss his tall tales as witchcraft or heresy.

The Desert and Madness

Being chased by mobs and fighting devils, and being paranoid and delusional echo the ramblings of schizophrenics. Was Antony schizophrenic? Of course, in ancient Christianity, madness was not medicalized, so this term might not even be appropriate. However, today one might wonder about Antony's sanity. Dr. Daniel Paul Schreber (1903/2000)—in his *Memoir of My Nervous Illness*—describes descents into madness. Not unlike Antony, Schreber writes about gods and monsters, being paranoid and engaging in delusional thinking.

Thomas Merton (1958) exclaims: "the desert is the country of madness" (p. 6) and psyche contains a desert-like madness. The search for God is this madness. It is also the case that the desert is a place where one might go mad. One wonders whether Jesus' visions in the desert were a descent into madness. Albert Schweitzer (1913), from a psychiatric point of view, argued that Jesus could have suffered from schizophrenia. It is written that Jesus walked on water, resurrected Lazarus, and talked to God. Schizophrenics often suffer delusions and think that God talks to them, or that they are God, or that they can perform miracles.

Myth, Madness and Archetypes

It is precisely *because of* the mythological aspect of religions that draw people into these stories. Jung did groundbreaking work on the mythological and archetypal nature of religion. Jung claimed that religion taps into archetypes—cross-cultural images—that are collectively unconscious. For Jung the collective unconscious is not the personal unconscious, as it was for Freud. The collective unconscious is an impersonal force that interpenetrates cultures across history. Archetypal images, say, of walking on the backs of crocodiles tap into an impersonal collective unconscious across space and time and history.

Jung's *Red Book*: The Collective Unconscious and Religion

Jung's (2009) *Red Book* was written when he suffered a psychotic break after a falling-out with Freud. Jung's book includes his artwork, paintings and drawings of dragons, monsters, mandalas. The images in the *Red Book* –Jung claims— are archetypal. The driving questions here are: is it possible that Schreber, Jung, Antony and Jesus expressed archetypal patterns that resonate across time and space? Is this the root of religious consciousness, one might wonder? How strangely serendipitous it is that these three figures lived in different times and places and yet all tapped into similar imagery.

One Agathon—who lived around the 3rd century CE—(cited in Ward, 1975) said: " It was said of Abba Agathon that for three years he lived with a stone in his mouth, until he had learnt to keep silence" (p. 22). Jung wrote about the importance of stones as archetypes. Stones had a special place in Jung's heart. He often meditated sitting on a large stone outside of his home. Stones are personified for Jung, as they were for Gaston Bachelard (2002) the French philosopher who wrote about the importance of stones and rocks as animate objects.

Bachelard argued that the earth is animate; the earth is composed of matter and so too is the imagination. The imagination is matter—just like the earth— because sentient beings and non-sentient things are made from the same stuff of the universe. Bachelard (2002) was no stranger to Jung.

Second Meditation: An Ecology of Death

Matthew von Umwerth (2005) writes meticulously about Freud's essay "On Transience." Von Umwerth (2005) tells us that Freud writes about a walk he takes with two friends—perhaps fictionalized, perhaps not. Von Umwerth explains that these two friends to which Freud refers were Andreas Lou-Salome, champion of psychoanalysis, and Rainer Maria Rilke, the hopelessly depressed poet. Against the horrors of war, Freud writes about how Lou-Salome and Rilke felt about the notion of transience. Lou-Salome and Rilke both felt that transience—that life is but a fleeting moment in time—was little more than depressing. If life is nothing more than a transient state of being, what is the point? Both Lou-Salome and Rilke longed for immortality. Longing for immortality, Freud called "a revolt... against mourning" (p. 219, cited in Von Umwerth, 2005). Freud writes that longing for immortality "is a product of our wishes" (in von Umwerth, 2005, p. 216) and the inability to go with the flow that is life that ends with death. The inability to accept that we die, for Freud, is highly problematic; it is a form of denial.

Freud argues that there are two ways of approaching transience: "despondency" or "rebellion" (p. 215, cited in Von Umwerth, 2005). Transience, for Freud, should not lead to despondency but to urgency. The rebellion about which Freud writes concerns time. The urgency of time is something about which we might rebel; for, without a deadline—without the deadline that is death—little would be accomplished. Transience, for Freud, is a gift, not a curse. Transience, therefore, is not something that one should be depressed about. One should, instead, see it as site of urgency.

An ecology of death—what I call *The Second Meditation*—entails the cyclical nature of life. For everything there is a season. Turn, turn, turn. So goes the Biblical verse. Ecology suggests that things are cyclical, not linear. Every day we die a little—this is also written in the story of Antony—as told through the mouthpiece of Athanasius (1980), drawing on the Christian Scriptures "I die daily" (p. 45). Pre-Socratic Greek philosopher Empedocles put it this way: there is "perpetual life in death and death in life" (cited in Marshall, 1891, p. 73). Death—going back to the earth, serves as nourishment for other creatures who then "live on"—as Derrida might put it. The cycle of rebirth is one that is ecological. Rebirth does not literally mean being resurrected—so that one might go to heaven—but, rather, resurrection could figuratively mean becoming nourishment for other creatures.

Dirt—ecologists tell us—is profoundly filled with life. The system of decay is profound; it is even alchemical. After decay, the body enters into yet another form and yet another—finally entering into what Edward Casey (1998) calls "the void"—which is a word early on in Genesis. The void—as an idea—also appears in multitudinous writings –Casey reports—such as Chang Tzu; it appears in Mayan texts and in the Upanishads (1998, p. 19). In pre-Socratic philosophy the void appears in the writings of Lucretius (2007) and Epicurus (2019), for example.

Interestingly, Casey (1998) points out that for orthodox Jews and fundamentalist Christians "The void is evaded, and in its stead we find a proliferation of cosmogonically significant places [emphasized in daily religious practice] each of which is essential to the progress of the narrative of creation" (p. 14). Importantly, Casey asks: "Does this narrativized proliferation of places betray an effort to paper over the abyss of the void" (p. 14)? The thought of the void creates terror and even perhaps what Freud calls "despondency." If our death is disappearance into nothingness—the void—what is the point of life?

Edward Casey (1998) is right to point out that progressive narratives—that erase the void—"paper over" (p. 14) what is unthinkable, and in this case, endings. John Donne's famous poem *Death Be Not Proud* is really about the "death of death," as David Marno (2016, p. 5) puts it. "What makes "Death be not Proud" a unique poem… is its seemingly unqualified triumph. At the end of the poem, the speaker announces the Death of Death and by implication his faith in the resurrection" (Marno, 2016, p. 5). Resurrection is yet another a way to "paper over," in Casey's (1998, p. 14) words, "the void" (p. 14).

Papering over the void and avoiding what one would rather not think about is not only a problem for religious people. Sandeep Jauhar (2008)—who writes from the perspective of a medical intern—states, "Though I was almost halfway through residency, I still wasn't sure whether I even *believed* in intensive care" (p. 243). Jauhar (2008) argues that

> In the ICU, doctors were prone to an irrational compulsion to do something—anything—no matter how futile or inane…. The stakes were high, the patients were sick, and you were supposed to act with conviction, even if there was no basis for it. And the therapies were hardly benign. Ventilators caused pneumonia, intravenous pressors caused arrhythmias, central lines caused infections and collapsed lungs, bed confinement caused blood clots and deconditioning… in the ICU sometimes it was impossible to do no harm. (p. 243)

ICUs keep people in a state of mythical suspension. Letting someone die—when life is no longer sustainable—is kinder than putting people on machines. Jauhar (2008) intimates that when life is no longer sustainable, the ICU is a place of cruelty (here patients are intubated, unconscious, or in comas). To die with dignity—when quality of life is gone—means letting someone die. The irony here is that—in my experience as a hospital chaplain—it is religious fundamentalists (mostly) who want to continue artificially keeping someone alive on machines, when there is no hope for any quality of life. And yet, religious fundamentalists are the same people, who are strongly opposed to vaccines—which are proven safe and efficacious—in the midst of a pandemic. What is the difference between a vaccine—an artificial treatment—and being intubated in an ICU?

My roles as scholar, teacher and hospital chaplain have led me to better understand that it is the very nature of belief, in and of itself, the reification of the idea of belief, that is the root cause of many problems in both education and the work that I do as a hospital chaplain. C.S. Peirce's (1877) in *Fixation of Belief* argues that any "fixation of belief," habitual or routine thought and behavior lead to "cruelties... [and] atrocities of the most horrible kind" (p. 20). Peirce intimates that it is easy to "fix" one's beliefs because one does not have to think. (Unthought) belief leads to "cheap pleasure which will not be followed by the least disappointment" (pp. 16-17). What Peirce calls "cheap pleasure" is the equivalent to what Dietrich Bonhoeffer called cheap grace. Grace is cheapened by trite consolations, and simple answers to complex theological dilemmas. Pierce compares a person with fixed beliefs to an ostrich who "buries its head in the sand as danger approaches... It hides the danger, and calmly says there is no danger" (p. 17).

The task, Peirce argues, is to break through that which is reified. Peirce argued that it is better to live in a state of doubt than lie to oneself. Peirce (1877) proclaims: "There must be a real and living doubt" (p. 14) to cut through what Dewey called everyday "hum drum" or what Avital Ronell (2002) boldly calls "stupidity." Rather, Peirce points out that we should embrace doubt, and learn to live with being uncomfortable. Challenges to the taken-for-granted come with some resistance, of course; but these (psychological) resistances need to be broken through. Peirce (1877) states that "doubt is an uneasy and dissatisfied state" (p. 12). It is far more difficult to live in a state of doubt than to live with "fixed beliefs."

Scholars, teachers and those who work in pastoral care must be able to continually question our own presuppositions and be willing to critique our own (unthought) belief systems. Marx (1976) once said that we need to engage in the "ruthless critique of everything"—including our own faulty thinking, our own "stupidities" (Ronell, 2002).

Reversing Descartes' Meditations

Although I modeled this introduction after Descartes's *Meditations*, I reverse his positions. Descartes began in doubt. That was a good start. The problem is that he ended in certainty. Peirce, contrarily, had it right. Instead of giving up doubt—in the quest for certainty—we need to live in a continual state of doubt. Thomas Merton (1998) lived in this continual state of doubt, even at the moment he took his vows. The *Meditations*—that I have written to introduce this book—begin and end in doubt. My aim in this book is not to search for certainties or even come to conclusions. This book is not about solutions. It is about raising questions.

When I began this book—as I mentioned earlier—it was not going to be about the pandemic. I started writing this book in 2018. There was no pandemic in 2018. And then the world suddenly changed. We have been thrown into utter upheaval and now more than ever "fixed beliefs" as Peirce puts it or reified ideas, as Adorno (2008) puts it, have been thrown into doubt. What disasters ask of us is perhaps beyond our capabilities. And it is to this beyond-ness—of all—certainty—that needs to be reconceptualized. The ever-shifting ground beneath our feet might cause existential nausea, but that is where we are historically. There is no going back behind the pandemic; there will be no normal to return to because nothing was ever normal to begin with.

Study and Theory: An Economy of Words

William Pinar (2009) writes about what he calls a "phenomenology of study" (p. 65). Here, he argues that "[s]tudy does not just yield new "information," it restructures one's subjectivity, animating and focusing one's engagement with the world" (p. 65). Being a scholar, teacher and chaplain demand study, solitude and indeed "focus," what Thomas Merton called "Inner discipline" (Merton, 2007 p. 73). David Marno (2016) calls for a "phenomenology of holy attention" (p. 5).

Being a scholar, teacher and chaplain requires one to retreat—at times—to contemplate, to meditate. Merton (1966) argues: "the contemplative life... must not be construed as an escape from time and matter, from social responsibility and from the life of sense, but rather as an advance into solitude and the desert" (p. 16). This too is Pinar's (2009) claim: scholars should live "passionate lives in public service." Contemplation, retreat and meditation go hand-in-glove with engagement in public service, especially in the midst of a pandemic.

Benedicta Ward (1975) remarks that the desert fathers (and mothers) exercised a "great economy of words" (p. xxii). As a chaplain an "economy of words" (Ward, 1975, p. xxii)—rather than idle chatter—allows spaces of grief to open and to be expressed. It is not the place of the chaplain to speak for others. Others' pain is a living text of alterity. Opening a space for others to speak or not requires a disciplined silence on the part of chaplains. "The last clinical imperative"—as Lacanian psychoanalyst Rob Weatherhill (1998, p. 184-185) put it—means embracing "the rigour of the real" (p. 185)—that death is death.

A chaplain must—as Nicholas Diat (2019) might say—"know how to lose [her/his] time for the sick" (p. 61). Giving up one's time for the death of the Other is an ethical imperative. Death comes in its own time. We must wait alongside grieving families. Henri Nouwen (2010) says, "Let us not diminish the power of waiting" (p. 72). Waiting for death is not easy. Waiting while the doctor breaks the bad news is not easy. Waiting is a form of meditation; It is a broken meditation on nothingness. Education is also a form of a broken meditation—especially now, during this horrific pandemic. Education—demands change—to reflect what it is we are experiencing right now. To pretend that nothing is happening, to carry on in the classroom as if the world does not matter, is irresponsible and unethical.

John Chryssavgis (2002) remarks that "many of them [the desert monastics] were lettered: Aresenius, Basil, Evagrius, and Cassian" (p. 77). Interestingly, Chryssavgis (2002) comments that these monks felt that "secular education always remained insufficient without ascetic depth [education was]... unfulfilled without the spiritual content" (p. 77). There is some debate about whether Antony—considered the father of monasticism—was literate or not (Harmless, 2004). It is perhaps myth that Antony did not read or write—according to Harmless (2004). Many commentators make the claim that Antony was illiterate. But Harmless (2004) reveals letters that are attributed to Antony. Perhaps he wrote them, perhaps not. Perhaps Antony did not exist at all. He did seem a creature out of myth, slaying dragons and walking on top of crocodiles. The upshot here is that education becomes empty without engagement with the Real, with or without "spiritual content" (Chryssavgis, 2002, p. 77). Being lettered—as were many of the desert fathers and mothers—is important, no doubt. Being educated, though, might mean something different. One can still be educated—confronting the

Real—without being lettered. However, a good university education, still, has meaning, in a seemingly meaningless universe.

The desert monastics encourage asceticism: "Go sit in your cell, and your cell will teach you everything" (attributed to one Abbas Moses, cited in Mayers, 1996). For Antony, the tomb was his cell. Analytic philosopher Ludwig Wittgenstein (1984)—at a certain time in his life—lived in a hut—much like a tomb or cell—in order to write. Like Antony, Wittgenstein (1984) proclaimed that one does not have to travel to go down deep—philosophically speaking (see *Culture and Value*). Travel does not necessarily make one wise.

Carlo Carretto (2002) reminds: "it was Thomas Merton who taught us that solitude is not simply a matter of geography" (p. x). No matter where one finds oneself—in a cell, a cave, a busy hospital emergency room, or on a desert landscape—psychic space and solitude are possible. We must allow the Other to go into that psychic space, especially in the midst of disaster.

Thomas Merton (2019) says the desert fathers embraced *"Anachoresis-* solitude" (p. 75). Plotinus' maxim: "alone with the Alone," *solus ad Solum* (p. 75) Merton says "does not exclude charity" (p. 75). Charity means the capacity to give up one's time for those who are in the midst of a tragedy. Charity—a taken-for-granted concept—might be more akin to hospitality—in the way that Derrida (2000) used the term. Hospitality is, indeed, a form of charity, a giving up of oneself for the Other. In fact, charity is an ancient concept that monastics used meaning taking care of the sick. One desert father named Arsenius stated, "At least go and visit the sick for that is also charity" (p. 16, in Ward, 1975). One Ammonas said: "Abba Agathon said, "If I could meet a leper, give him my body and take his... "that would be perfect charity" (p. 24, in Ward, 1975). The pandemic has made chaplaincy all the more challenging and dangerous. Doubt. We don't know what we are doing. At the beginning of the covid pandemic nobody knew what they were doing, medical staff included. There was not yet a vaccine. There was nothing. The medical staff and chaplains were blindly wading through mine fields. As Ellsberg (2018) states "there are risks to be faced by those who travel without maps" (p. 38). We had no maps. It was, indeed, a frightening time.

Third Meditation

Meditation, doubt and unbearable stories are the topic at hand. Unbearable stories are those that readers cannot bear to read; unbearable stories are those that writers cannot bear to write. However, in the very act of reading unbearable stories we become co-writers in the texts at hand.

Curriculum-writ-large concerns educative experiences outside the formal walls of the schoolhouse. This book is mainly about educative experiences outside of formal institutions. At this current juncture in history unbearable stories surround us. Nothing makes sense in this age of Covid-19.

This book is an attempt at archivization of that which is impossible to archive. The Greek concept *arche,* according to John Marshall (1891), means "the originative principle" (p. 10). For Derrida, this is no "originative principle." There is no original unbearable story; the question of where covid began is not important. The fact of the matter is that covid is here, now.

Unbearable stories are webbed within the memory of other unbearable stories and those unbearable stories are yet webbed yet again within other unbearable stories. Stories are about the self in relation to the Other in the context of history and culture. History is made of that which is unbearable. Wars, plagues, death and destruction, violence and pandemics are the stuff of history. Our educations cannot exclude the curriculum-writ large of these unbearable histories.

Thomas Merton (1964) proclaims: "one of the awful facts of our age is the evidence that it is stricken to the very core of its being by the presence of the unspeakable" (p. 5). Merton's over-arching unspeakable theology is that God's grace is found in absence; God's mercy is found in silence. When confronting unspeakable trauma, God's absence and silence puzzles—says Merton.

Absence, doubt, silence. Whether one is religious or not, Merton speaks profoundly; he speaks—presciently- to an era he did not live through—the covid era. Still his words are relevant today. Silence in the face of death is something one must confront. Doubt about the future, if there is to be one at all, troubles. Absence of those who have perished pains. We are left with the questions: why? Why now? Why my loved one? Why me? There are no answers or words of consolation in the face of death, especially when death and suffering could have been prevented.

Judith Butler (2020) writes about living in precarious times. Butler (2020) comments that what gets represented—about precarious times—(and here I will add the particular case of the era of covid-19) is controlled by "the boundaries that constitute what will and will not appear within public life, the limits of a publicly acknowledged field of appearance" (p. xix). What it is that we see on television and social media are controlled and manipulated. Most do not have first-hand access to what goes on inside of hospitals on covid wards. The gruesome deaths and realities that people suffer when they no longer have any sustainable life left or hope for survival remain mostly absent from public view. Television sanitizes end of life catastrophes on covid wards. As time passes, the public sees little about the way in which covid plays out in hospitals. The public, therefore, is left in a blank space—not knowing what is going on. This blank space does not help inform the public and it indeed shapes how people perceive—or do not perceive—this catastrophe. Educating the public is the heart and soul of what I do: this book is a testimony to public education. This book is an attempt to educate the public not only about covid, but it is also a testimony to the responsibility educators have to tell the stories that need to be told, even if they are unbearable.

I am a first-hand witness to covid deaths—working on covid wards as a hospital chaplain. I feel that it is my duty and responsibility to attempt to untangle and educate the public in the only way I know how, through words, through writing. But this book is not about the literalness of death and dying. This book is an attempt to think through—philosophically, theologically, culturally, psychoanalytically, politically—the unfolding catastrophe of covid.

In order to educate the public, "precarious" stories—as Judith Butler (2020) puts it—need to be unpacked in ways that get at what it is that is still and perhaps always will be beyond understanding. We are too close historically to understand what is happening to us, but it is this impossible—and precarious—task I undertake.

Unbearable stories in this book are theorized through curriculum studies, theology, philosophy, memoir, literary fiction, biography and autobiography and memoir. I come at this project in an interdisciplinary fashion so as not to simplify or reduce the complexities of the history we are living through. This is a multidisciplinary archive. It is an unending archive. It is an archive, too, that is perspectival. I do not pretend to come at this from a God's eye view. I come at this through my perspective and take responsibility for that perspective. What I see and what I say are always already partial.

Woven throughout the book, I include some stories from the frontlines—with boots on the ground—as a hospital chaplain. I also tell the tale of my experiences in the professoriate, witnessing the tragic no-response in a Republican strong-hold. I come to no conclusion at the close of the book. I offer no consolation. This is not a book about lessons to be learned or lessons to teach. In the face of needless suffering and needless deaths, no didactics are at hand. Nothing good comes from what is terrible. There is no light at the end of the tunnel. There are no happy endings to be had. My intellectual work over the years has had a consistent theme: never gloss over that which is unthinkable.

Chapter Outlines

Chapter One concerns clinical narrative and its stultification. This chapter problematizes clinical case studies, romantic science and medical anthropology. Here, I focus on Michel Foucault's (1994) *The Birth of the Clinic*, A.R. Luria's (2002) *The Man with the Shattered World*, and medical anthropologist Arthur Frank's (1997) *The Wounded Storyteller*. Clinical case studies, romantic science and medical anthropology—as forms of narrative—are troubled. All three genres serve to stultify unbearable stories. The clinical narrative fails because it serves to sanitize and gloss over unbearable stories.

Chapter Two concerns what is termed speculative fabulation and unbearable stories. This chapter explores the notion of speculative fabulation drawing on Donna Haraway (2001). It is noted that speculative fabulation allows for the "wildness" of the unbearable story to be told without domestication. Speculation—in the philosophical sense—is unpacked to better understand the historicity of this term. Fabulation—as a concept—is also teased out so as to clarify what this might mean in the context of unbearable stories. The argument in this chapter is that speculation is shot through with fantasy and fabulation (which I argue are puzzles of perception.) Fantasy and perception together form the way in which unbearable stories are told and perhaps understood.

Chapter Three explores Jacques Derrida's (1976; 1978; 1986; 1996) unwieldy concepts of the archive, the trace and differance in order to deconstruct speculative fabulation. Deferred and delayed meaning—as Derrida (1986; 1996) puts it—are in the service of the archivization of memory and history. The elusiveness of the trace—as a concept—thickens the theorization of unbearable stories. Derrida's three concepts are architectonically built upon the notion of speculative fabulation as defined in Chapter Two. Together, speculative fabulation and Derrida's three concepts help to unpack the telling of unbearable stories.

Chapter Four concerns Thomas Merton's (1966) crisis of the unspeakable. Merton approaches theological crises without gloss or consolation. Like Derrida, Merton addresses what cannot be addressed by utilizing paradoxes or aporias. For Merton, God's absence is grace; God's silence is mercy. These theological propositions lure us into predicaments that puzzle. This chapter explores unspeakable theology as a puzzle and a puzzlement. The theoretical concepts in Chapters One, two and three will be interwoven throughout the remainder of the book to help unpack the unbearable stories at hand.

Chapter Five examines Terry Tempest Williams' (2001) *Refuge*, Joan Didion's (2005) *The Year of Magical Thinking* and Derrick Jensen's (2000) *Language Older than words*. These unbearable stories are explored through the theoretical lens of speculative fabulation and deepened by Derrida's concepts of differance, the archive and the trace. This chapter explores compounded grief of death, child abuse and rape. These stories, although not directly related to covid-19, help us to better articulate the ways in which mourning and grief get expressed, or not, through a variety of lenses and perspectives.

Chapter Six examines Anton Boisen's (1952) *The Exploration of the Inner World*, Louise DeSalvo's (2018) *The House of Early Sorrows*, and John Gunther's (1998) *Death Be Not Proud*. All three stories are, in their own way, unbearable. Here, mental breakdown, incest, the death of a child are unpacked. Like the previous chapter, the stories in this chapter are not directly related to covid-19 but they help us to better grapple with the way in which people attempt to cope with, or not, personal tragedies.

Chapter Seven begins by looking at Camus' (1995) autobiographical novel, *The First Man* to better understand how his later fiction is shot through with his biographic situation. I argue in this chapter that one cannot understand Camus' fiction—in a deeper sense—if one is not familiar with Camus' early childhood. After situating Camus biographically, I look at Camus' (1989) *The Stranger* and Camus' (1948) *The Plague*. Camus' novels uncannily resonate with the current catastrophe that is covid.

Chapter Eight examines a variety of Michel Serres' (2007; 1995; 2000; 1991) texts including *The Parasite, Genesis, The Birth of Physics* and *Rome: The Book of Foundations*. Serres' writings—uncannily—deal with the history of plagues throughout the ancient world. What Serres has to say about plagues—historically—has relevance to what we are experiencing currently with covid-19. Serres is a philosopher of science; thus, his work deals with such scientific and philosophical concepts as turbulence, noise, the clinamen and the swerve. These concepts might help us to better articulate—in a phenomenological and existential way—what it is like to experience living through a pandemic.

Notes

1. The concept of meditation was used by Descartes to veil his work on reason in theological terms in an effort to straddle theology and the scientific study of knowledge. It could be the case that Descartes did this in an effort to avoid persecution by the Church.

2. Religion and theology are two separate concepts. As I see it, religion, generally speaking, concerns dogma and the practices of ritual. Theology concerns systematic theoretical conceptualization of the divine, or the holy.
3. There were many apocalyptic texts that were excluded from the Bible. Stories of the apocalypse were a popular genre before the bible was codified. Interestingly enough, contemporary science fiction seems obsessed with stories of the apocalypse. Science fiction and religion—uncannily—share certain characteristics.
4. Biblical scholars sometimes utilize what is referred to as the historical-critical method to study ancient texts. Here scholars look for patterns, genres, styles of writing and possible historical events that undergird their theories. However, no one knows for certain who wrote what when. Biblical scholars use what is called source theory (e.g., sources refer to different groups of writers such as the P source, because of similar patterns of writing styles). The P source (the Priestly source), for example, is attributed to genealogical passages (the list of begats in the Hebrew Scriptures) or passages that order things (on the first day, on the second day etc., God created the world and so forth). The bible was redacted; books were written and organized by many—about whom we have little, if any, information. The bible was not put together in a linear fashion. Books that are historically younger were actually placed at the end of, say, the Hebrew Scriptures, while older books were placed first (i.e. the book of Genesis was not, in fact, the first book—historically—in the Hebrew Scriptures.) Genesis was probably the last book in the Pentateuch. Some of the letters of Paul are not—in fact—Paul's but are attributed to others. The Book of Isaiah is thought to be written by different people because patterns in the text point to style differences that might indicate that there were, in fact, several Isaiahs, not one. Some of the passages in the bible are based on historical events—such as a flood, or perhaps, floods. However, many bible texts are mythological. There is debate whether Moses was a real person. We know that many were called sons of God, although Jesus today is referred to as the son of God. There were many people named Jesus as well. And crucifixions were common. One thing is clear: scholars have come to little consensus on what—in the biblical texts—is historically accurate or whether events happened at all. This gets further complicated by biblical translations, especially after the Reformation in the 1600s. Moreover, there were many competing books—alongside the bible—such as the Gnostic Gospels—that were excluded from the biblical

canon because they were deemed heretical. Hermeneutics—the study of interpretation—emerged as a systematic theological field of study because of these competing debates. There is one thing, however, that academic biblical scholars agree upon: a literal reading of the bible is not tenable. However, fundamentalists interpret the bible literally, believing that, for example, God wrote the bible, or that Moses wrote the first five books of the bible, or that the book of Revelation is based on real predictions of the future.

5. That death is not beautiful is a reference to the title of a 1997 film about the Holocaust *Life is Beautiful*. The title of this Holocaust film needs to be troubled because life was not beautiful during the Holocaust, nor was death. That title strikes me as unethical, for it serves to gloss over the horror of the Holocaust. I have also made these points elsewhere (see Morris, 2001).

1

Clinical Narratives and Stultification

All medical personnel chart on their patients. Charts are computerized databases. Chart notes are legal documents. Chart notes are clinical; the problem is this: chart notes are stultifying. Physicians chart diagnoses and prognoses, nurses chart dispensed medicines, social workers chart discharge plans, and chaplains chart spiritual *outcomes*?! What exactly is a spiritual outcome? Charting is a way of quantifying the *productivity* of the chaplain. Productivity translates in the following way: how many patients per hour did the chaplain visit? Administrators check chart notes for quality assurance.

Charting is about checklists. All the boxes must be checked off appropriately. Who called the chaplain? How many family members did the chaplain visit? Emotions of patients noted. Box one is fear, box two is anxiety, and box three is depression. The religion of the patient is noted. The spiritual outcome is also on this checklist.

Baptism—a ritual—is performed by all chaplains if requested, no matter their own tradition. If baptism is performed, it is checked off in a box on the medical chart. There is but little space for any narrative. The narrative chaplains write is limited to number of words; subjective statements get excised from the record so as to avoid lawsuits. Chaplain narratives must sound clinical; they must be filled with meaningless jargon. Chart notes must read as if they were written by a computer programmer.

A typical example of a chaplain's chart notes reads as follows: "The chaplain arrived on scene at 1300 hours. The chaplain engaged in a brief life review with the patient. The patient was a victim of a gunshot wound. The patient has two siblings who were also shot at the scene. The patient's emotional response was incongruent to the situation. The patient's affect was flat. The patient suffers from compounded grief as he is experiencing multiple losses, as his mother died from a gunshot wound and his father was stabbed. The chaplain offered a ministry of presence and the family was appreciative."

Chart notes must be concise, objective, clear and formulaic. No interpretations are permitted. Just the facts. The chaplain's chart notes read like a police report and are, in fact, considered legal documents. James Hillman (1983) puts it this way: "A clinician is supposed to note the way stories are told" (p. 15). Verbatim accounts—of patients' stories—are expected. But is there any way to really write a verbatim account? In the emergency room, there is a lot going on at once. Emergency rooms are full of chaos. Chaplains who report to the emergency room for a trauma can, in no way, report the way things happened—exactly, that is, verbatim. Things get left out, forgotten, and misunderstood. Objectivity is impossible.

Chaplains are considered clinicians. How is chaplaincy clinical? How is a patients' narrative clinical—especially when it concerns issues of heart, emotions and spirituality? The patient's emotional and spiritual lives are messy, incoherent, anguished, angry, violent. James Hillman (1983) remarks, "There are no bare events, plain facts, simple data—or rather this too is an archetypal fantasy" (p. 23). Patients in hospitals are usually traumatized, terrified, sometimes they have no words to describe what they are experiencing. To report—from the chaplain's perspective—the traumatized patient's story in clinical language, sterile language, actually serves as an injustice to the patient who wants to tell her story.

Those who have unbearable stories to tell—in this context, in the case of covid-19—are so utterly traumatized that they cannot even speak. By the time the chaplain arrives, the patient is nearing death, on a ventilator and unconscious. Families cannot visit covid patients, so chaplains counsel them over the phone or on the computer screen through web ex technology. Families cannot visit covid patients in most hospitals because the risk of infection is too high. Their last visit with their loved one is usually via technology on a computer screen. The families want to see their loved one, but what they see is probably not what they thought they would to see. What they see—through enclosed glass windows—are those who are hooked up to machines, unconscious and nearing death. How to chart this kind of unspeakable trauma? Chart note reads: "Mother screamed on phone when chaplain called." "Family member hung up on doctor when he called to report the bad news that covid patient was about to die." "Wife of covid patient cannot believe what she sees as the computer screen and camera is held up to the glass outside of the patient's room." "Wife of dying husband on ventilator utters two words: "That's sad."

How to chart that? How to chart the unsaid, the unthinkable. The scream. Hanging up on the doctor. The rage. The horror. Existential crisis? Check a box. Patient died. Check a box. Charting unbearable stories as if they are police reports helps no one.

Chaplains are trained by writing up what are termed "verbatims." The chaplain is supposed to write down verbatim conversations that she had with the patients and families. Each sentence is marked by a number; as if the number quantifies and clarifies what is said. Part of the problem is that by the time the chaplain sits down to write up the "verbatim" half of the conversation is forgotten.

There are transference issues that get in the way of what the chaplain hears and what the chaplain wants to hear. What gets written down—in fact—is shot through with transference. Getting the story right is impossible. Fantasy and erasure, erosion of memory or embellishment—because of transference—makes verbatims impossible. The story the patient tells becomes partly the chaplain's projections. Nothing is what it seems and, in reality, all is subjective.

Verbatims are presented to the chaplain's supervisor for critique. Monday morning quarterbacking is of little use. It all seems too simple and clear-cut. Michel Foucault (1994), in *Birth of the Clinic,* speaks to these kinds of problems:

> The clinic—constantly praised for its empiricism, the modesty of its attention, and the care with which it silently lets things surface to the observing gaze without disturbing the discourse— owes its real importance to the fact that it is a reorganization in depth, not only of medical discourse, but of the very possibility of a discourse about disease. The *restraint* [emphasis in the original] of clinical discourse (its rejection of theory, its abandonment of systems, its lack of philosophy; all so proudly proclaimed by doctors) reflects the non-verbal conditions on the basis of which it can speak: the common structure that carves up and articulates what is seen and what is said. (p. xix)

The chaplain follows the medical model Foucault critiques here. The chaplain is supposed to engage in a clean and clear *empirical* evaluation of the patient's existential crisis, spiritual condition and emotional state. The empirical nature of the chaplain's evaluation is the first problem at hand. Empirical observation is highly problematic. The chaplain cannot be an objective observer. It is impossible. The chaplain sees what she wants to, edits unconsciously—and perhaps unwittingly—through avoidance, aversion, disgust, fear and anguish. Emotional reactions on the part of the chaplain have to be edited out of the chart notes. The "restraint" Foucault points to above is constricting and absolutely stultifying. The story the patient tells gets redacted as it is put it into a seemingly logical sequence of events that must fall within the bounds of acceptable clinical jargon.

Judith Butler (2016) writes about the way in which war is "framed" by embedded reporters in war zones. The way something is "framed" determines how we see—and interpret—things. Butler (2016) states: "we are being recruited into… a certain framing of reality, both its construction and interpretation" (p. xii). Like embedded reporters in war zones, physicians and chaplains are "embedded" in emergency rooms filled with chaos and confusion. How to write a clear cut, clinical chart note in the middle of chaos? The stultification of narrative—that is expected of both physician and chaplain—does a certain violence to the patient's story. The "frame" of the medical narrative is technical: it is filled with numbers, jargon and is formulaic. As Foucault (1994) puts it: "the reductive discourse of the doctor" (p. xi) serves to pretend that "seeing and saying are still one" (p. xi). Nothing about the patient is really revealed except numbers that designate the progress of the disease, the deterioration of the patient's condition is reflected on x-rays, CT scans and MRIs. But numbers sometimes get it wrong.

Medical charts are what Judith Butler (2016) calls "a strategy of containment" (p. xiii). Medicine and chaplaincy conceal what I would call a narrative of the real because the real is too messy to contain. Numbers are slippery. Cancer tests such as the CA-125 which is supposed to be a tumor marker for ovarian cancer are sometimes wrong, and this can have disastrous consequences for the patient. The CA-125 serves to contain the emotions of the patient. If your number is below 35, the CA-125 reveals a healthy patient. Year in and year out cancer patients have to have CA-125s. After year 5, the tests slow down. But the tests create tremendous anxiety for patients; they also can re-traumatize patients. These tests are constant reminders that all is not well with the body; at any time, cancer can recur. And for ovarian cancer patients, this is especially bad. Not many survive the recurrence of ovarian cancer. And 70 % of all ovarian cancer patients will suffer from recurrence.

The patient's emotions—in the case of a high CA-125 reading—have fallen out of the "frame" of the medical chart. The frame of the medical chart—as Judith Butler (2016) might put it—serves as "polishing the surface of a melancholia whose rage must be contained, and often cannot" (p. xiii). Butler (2016) states that the function of the frame is to engage in "always throwing something away, always keeping something out" (p. xiii). The medical narrative that reads "poor prognosis" conceals the emotional horror at hand.

Adorno (2008) states that "common-sense thinking" demands a "frame of reference in which everything has its place" (p. 144). The problem is that some medical narratives have "no frame of reference." In the case of ovarian cancer—when the diagnosis is wrong—or Covid, when the "prognosis is grim" have "no frame of reference." Covid patients—once placed on the covid ward—have a grim prognosis. But what does "grim prognosis" contain? What story does this tell, or exclude?

The basic formula for chart notes turns on: who, what, where and when. This is very similar to police report writing. Foucault (1994) points out that what the clinical narrative does is "carves up" (p. xix) the narrative and "reorganizes" it. But more to the point, Foucault points out that this "reorganization" opens out to questions that go beyond mere report writing or medical charting. Clinical discourse that is held back by "restraint" altering patients' narratives to the point of being unrecognizable. What is said by the patients and what gets written down by the clinician are not the same. James Hillman (1983) puts it this way:

> Case history as factual history, a true account... is a fiction in the sense of a fabrication, a lie. But it is only a lie when it claims literal truth.... Freud found that he was not recording a true account of historical events, but fantasies of events as if they had actually happened. The material of a case history is not historical facts but psychological fantasies, the subjective stuff that is the proper domain of fiction. (p. 12)

The chaplain's chart notes, therefore, are subjective after all, no matter how cloaked in clinical jargon. The chaplain's chart notes are "psychological fantasies." The verbatims that are brought back to the supervisor are not, in fact, verbatim. They are memories—shot through with fantasies, reversals, forgettings, if you will. What the chaplain thinks she remembers is probably not totally the case. There is no such thing as a verbatim.

I wonder whether the training of chaplains is misguided. Foucault questions "the very possibility of a discourse of disease" (1994, p. xix). Here too, I question the "very possibility of a discourse" of chaplaincy. The re-telling of the patient's story gets distorted, twisted and rewritten in ways that probably do not reflect the situation at hand. But does that make the chaplain's narrative useless? Not entirely. The chaplain's chart notes can give medical personnel a different angle on the patient's overall condition. But no matter how one approaches the problems at hand, the chaplain's narrative is "proper to the domain of fiction" as Hillman (1983, p. 12) points out.

Freud felt that case histories were useful not in getting the facts right, but in how the patient made use of the story. Even if a childhood memory is completely mis-remembered, or made up, fabricated, it matters little. Freud argued that what matters is what the patient does with the material in the analysis. How does the patient use the analysis in the life that is to-come? But in the case of medical chart notes—for the chaplain or physician—the patient never sees these notes. So, for the patient they serve no purpose. These chart notes cannot be put to use. A patient can see test results, perhaps. But of what use are numbers?

The chaplain's verbatim, like the physician's narrative, as Foucault points out, "rejects theory" and "lacks philosophy" (1994 p. xix). Chart notes are hardly theoretical or philosophical. Perhaps during Freud's lifetime, case studies were amenable to theory and philosophy. Certainly, Freud's case studies are both theoretical and philosophical. But case studies written up in hospitals today are not like Freud's. Literary flair, or philosophical musing, is prohibited.

Physicians' narratives all read the same way, as if they are carbon copies of the same stories over and over again. Their narratives are concise, no-nonsense legal documents. Their narratives erase the human; all is reduced to the disease. The patient becomes the disease. Is the physician writing a narrative about a person or about a disease?

The humanities have been driven out of medicine; this is a terrible problem in patient care. Physicians—when making rounds—spend more time pushing their computers down the hall, charting, than talking with patients. Now it is true that physicians complain about the increasing weight placed on charting. But this is the future of medicine.

Non-for-profit hospitals are no longer fiscally sustainable in a culture where health care is about the bottom line. For-profit hospitals are driven by the bottom line. For-profit hospitals are also McDonaldized. They standardize care; and minimize cost. The McDonaldization of for-profit hospitals have turned medicine into Ford factories. Productivity means that medical personnel see as many patients as possible in one hour. Health care has turned into an industry of increasing profits, while cutting corners.

The Pandemic Belies Emotional Containment

The pandemic began slowly, it seemed. And then it began to feel as if time sped up as the floors filled up with covid patients. One floor, two floors, three floors, and then covid patients began spilling out into the general hospital population. The electronic boards on the covid floors seemed to get bigger and bigger, more and more patients began dying. Chaplains were spending more and more time calling family members, dealing with death and trauma, trying to work technologies like web ex, and other forms of telehealth. Medical personnel began to panic; some died by suicide. Others became numb. In the third year of the pandemic, nurses began quitting; staff shortages are emerging everywhere. The profession cannot contain this pandemic's emotional fallout—no matter how neat and tidy the chart notes.

There seemed to be no time to understand what was happening. More and more covid patients began piling into the hospital. Death after death after death. At first medical personnel—the nurses with whom I built relations—seemed stunned, horrified, some broke down in tears. It was overwhelming to watch helplessly as medical personnel could do little to save patients; it was exhausting for chaplains to try to pick up the pieces of broken lives.

And then there was silence. A lot of silence. How to chart these horrors? Emotional exhaustion does not allow one to process seeing so much death; the hospital felt like a war zone. These horrors cannot be processed immediately, if at all. When covid vaccines became available, chaplains were used less and less. Deaths decreased, floors opened up to the general hospital population, and finally chaplains were put on furlough. Until things got worse. In year two, covid-19 morphed into the delta variant and then things got bad again. Chaplains were called back to duty. And then again—after some time had passed—there was a lull, chaplains were let go again. Until omicron hit in the Spring of 2022. Once again chaplains were called back to duty and now things seemed to be even worse than the first year of covid, while in the media the CDC was reporting that the effects of omicron were mild. But this turned out not to be the case for many. The numbers of dead nearing one million, just in the United States alone. That should give us pause. The continual reporting of the numbers of deaths on television seemed to belie the horrors of the actual reality of death. Numbers numb: they become meaningless in the face of the reality of death. Numbers are not people. Numbers are symptoms of the clinical gone wrong. The numbers do not tell the stories of the victims of this horrific virus.

Foucault (1994) remarks that with the "birth of the clinic" medicine had become likened to a taxonomy of the body. Foucault states:

> Before it is removed from the density of the body, disease is given an organization, hierarchized into families, genera, and species.... But at a deeper level... classificatory medicine presupposes a Certain "configuration" of disease.... Just as the genealogical tree. (p. 4)

Chart notes are like "configurations," encyclopedic entries into a vast network of meaningless jargon. Time of death. Patient died. Call it. That is what the medical team hears when the patient no longer has a heartbeat after a code blue. The management of death seemed factory-like. The documentation of the funeral arrangements, the arrival of the undertaker, the body delivered to the morgue, the time the death was *called*. Call it. Patient coded. Jargon, meaningless and cold. Code blue. Patient died. Call it. The undertaker. The morgue. Over and over again. One after the next. McDonaldization. The Fordist model of the for-profit hospital.

Reading the log book at the morgue was particularly telling; something most are not privy to. Mrs. X Covid. Mr. Z Covid. Mrs Y Covid. Dates were scribbled after the names of the dead. After covid patients were wrapped *twice* in plastic—because they were still contagious even after death—they were (literally) tossed into refrigerated drawers. I remember hearing the thud of a body hitting the bottom of the refrigerator door and the feet sticking out. The nurses had to find a way to make the feet fit into the refrigerator. Gruesome, indeed. The routinization of tossing bodies into refrigerator drawers seemed like something out of a horror movie. Indeed, death became routinized.

The bodies had to stay in refrigerated drawers for forty-eight hours before transporting them to the morgue because they were still contagious. So the bodies piled up. And then came the refrigerated trucks where bodies just got piled up even higher. Morgues could not keep up with the corpses. The morgue logbook read like a catalog of death. Turning the pages of the logbook I was stunned by the sheer coldness of this routine. I watched as doctors and nurses moved dead bodies from covid wards covered over in two plastic bags—over and over again—from patient rooms to the morgue. One patient died, another one moved in the very same room. Then that patient died, the corpse was carted out; the next patient placed in the room. It was so macabre, so routinized, so banal. Medical personnel seemed totally numbed. Or so it seemed.

Nobody even blinked an eye. Another covid patient, another death. The faceless corpses covered up in white plastic bags, lumps of flesh dumped, or tossed into refrigerator drawers. It is still too soon to know how medical personnel will psychologically manage what they have witnessed. These are unbearable, faceless stories. Stories of the dead, without a face, an identity.

As I walk through the valley of the shadow of death became my mantra. Psalm 23. Silently saying it to myself, reciting it in empty hallways upon a family's request. But the family was not there. Just the chaplain, me, reciting Psalm 23 in an empty hallway. Meaningless. Words. During the lulls in-between covid surges, many medical personnel got furloughed. Most felt used and furious. Mbembe's (2019) term "necropolitics" began to take on real meaning.

These are the politics of death, covid and hospital profits. Who lives, who dies? Who decides? When ICUs are over capacity, those who seemingly do not matter, do not get the care that they need. The homeless, people of color, the poor, those without insurance, the elderly mattered less. Racism, classism and ageism all played a role in who lived and who died. Who got the care they needed and who did not. This is what "necropolitics" means, yet it still does not capture the heartache, confusion, depression, dissociation, silence, outrage and disorientation, rage that was part of what I have called covid collateral elsewhere. Although the political aspects of health care are crucial in understanding who lives and who dies, the covid pandemic cannot be reduced to political issues. Things are far more complicated than that.

This pandemic cannot be compared to anything; there are no precedents. The 1918 flu epidemic might be the closest thing we can compare this current catastrophe with; but still the covid pandemic is not the 1918 flu pandemic. Nonetheless, we do not have much to go on. In the beginning of the pandemic I recall nurses saying that all that they could do was throw cocktails of drugs at patients, hoping something would work. Treatments have improved since the beginning of the pandemic, but still the deaths are spiraling out of control, even in the third year of this pandemic.

Clinical Case Studies Versus Romantic Science

Oliver Sacks (1990; 1998) renowned neurologist describes heartless medical writing that pretends toward objectivity, resulting in the erasure of the human from medicine. Sacks (1990) opines: "modern medicine, increasingly, dismisses our existence,... reducing us to identical replicas" (p. 228). A heavily administered culture, or Adorno's (1966/2007) "administered world" (p. 20) —dictates what can be written into the medical charts—thereby constructing the acceptable stories which fit into formulaic "frame[s]" as Judith Butler (2016) puts it. Butler (2016) remarks, in her book on war, that "precarious" lives, are those who are deemed "ungrievable" (p. xix). Those who are marginalized are always-already left for dead, and therefore are not grieveable because they do not have cultural capital. In the hospital, those whose lives are "precarious" (p. 13) and "ungrievable" (p. xix) are the poor, people of color and the elderly as I mentioned earlier, or patients who are already known to the medical community as "drug seeking" "multi-substance" abusers and those who are "noncompliant." Blaming the victim is easy; being compassionate is not. These might be over- generalizations and perhaps they should be qualified, but these responses by medical personnel are more prevalent than not. The unvaccinated are the worst offenders of all. Health professionals are growing tired of taking care of the people who did not take care of themselves. The unvaccinated put health care workers' lives at risk; hence, resentment has become a topic of discussion especially in the third year of the pandemic. Medical professionals take an oath to do no harm. Whether resentment is or is not justified is not part of medical training. No matter how medical personnel feel about their patients, they must do no harm. Resentment or not. Judith Butler (2016) states:

> Ungrievable lives are those that cannot be lost, and cannot be destroyed, because they already inhabit a lost and destroyed zone; they are, ontologically, and from the start, already lost and destroyed. (p. xix)

Even before entering the doors of the emergency room, there are those patients whose lives are already "ungreivable" for these are the people nobody cares about, the homeless, drug addicts, the poor, people of color, immigrants. Nonetheless, medical personnel must treat everybody who comes through those emergency room doors, no matter who they are. But if patients seem to be self-destructive, if patients do harm to themselves, if patients are morbidly obese or unvaccinated, if patients are multi-substance abusers or drug seekers—medical personnel report—although they have to be objective that they are losing patience with their patients. The medical community is exhausted. Still, the oath to do no harm is the oath the medical community takes seriously; they live by this oath, regardless of losing patience. Although medical journals are filled with scientific papers on covid, on vaccines and possible treatments, it is not often that physicians write papers on their emotions. Nurses are more apt to report emotions in medical humanities journals, especially if they take a phenomenological perspective. These engendered documents reveal a culture of a continued crisis of masculinity. It is not considered professional (read masculine) to report on one's emotional responses, say, to the unvaccinated.

Oliver Sacks (1990) comments that papers in medical journals—read no differently from chart notes.

> One mulls over whole libraries of papers, couched in the "objective," style less style de rigueur in neurology; one's head buzzes with "facts," figures, lists, schedules, inventories, calculations, ratings, quotients, indices, statistics,... and proved in a manner which would have delighted the heart of Thomas Gradgrind. (p. 230)

Kafka's (1915) gatekeeper *Before the Law* describes even better the bureaucracy behind "facts," "figures" and "lists." Administrators are the gatekeepers before the law. The administrators put under surveillance all "facts" "figures" and "lists." The gatekeeper-administrator edits out emotion, eloquence, the seemingly subjective.

It is unfortunate that case studies—like those written by Freud (which read like works of literature) are not permissible today. Case studies—in the style of Freud, or Oliver Sacks—are nowhere to be found in chart notes. Writing up cases in any style "whatsoever" (Luc-Nancy, 1996) is not permissible in a highly administered (medical) culture.

Thus, without detailed narrative, perspective or interpretation, little is learned about the (human) patient. It should be noted, however, that Oliver Sacks does not wholly dismiss clinical case studies—as stultifying as they are; he argues that the clinical has a place in medicine but needs to be balanced out with more experiential—and human—representations of the patient.

Oliver Sacks is known for his published case studies, written for lay audiences. He engages in what is called *romantic science*, a phrase borrowed from A.R. Luria (1968; 2002), a renown Russian neuropsychologist. A.R. Luria wrote *stories* about his patients (not clinical taxonomies). Luria's most well-known case studies are *The Man with A Shattered World* (2002) and *The Mind of a Mnemonist* (1968).

Like Freud, Luria was a storyteller. Luria's (2002) *The Man With A Shattered World* is about a soldier who got shot in the head during WWII. Zazetsky—after getting shot—lost his memory, his identity; he lost his ability to read or write. Luria encouraged Zazetsky to try to write, even though he forgot how to write. After some time, Zazetsky could write a little, but he could not read what he had written. After more time, he began to understand some of what he had written. Zazetsky would re-write the same thing over and over again, forgetting what he had just rewritten. After some twenty years, though, Zazetsky was finally able to write his memoir and understand what he had written.

Luria's, (1968) *the Mind of A Mnemonist*, is about a patient with photographic memory. He could recall a long series of numbers backwards and forwards—for decades on end. This is a fascinating story of someone with a superhuman memory. What Luria demonstrates in these case studies are medical marvels that neurologists simply cannot explain.

Luria, Freud and Oliver Sacks wrote phenomenological and experiential case studies. Romantic science—as it is called—has unfortunately fallen out of fashion in the medical community. Today most case studies are clinical, stacked with numbers and jargon. Case studies—at least those written up in medical chart notes in a hospital—are formulaic.

Sacks compares Luria's work to Freud's (1993) *Three case histories: The "wolf man," the "rat man," and the psychotic doctor Schreber*. Unlike Luria or Sacks, Freud was the founder of psychoanalysis, but he was also a neurologist. Freud had no truck with the stultified methodologies of neurology. Freud knew that the mind was far more complicated than the scientific method could capture. But today, Freud has fallen out of fashion. Medicine has been colonized by quantification.

Oliver Sacks' popularizing of neurology—did not come without a price. Traditional neurologists tended to be highly critical of Sacks. However, there is a place for popularizing science. Lay persons could learn a great deal from reading Sacks' work; most lay persons cannot understand medical journals because they are written for a highly specialized readership.

Unlike romantic science, academic psychology has become medicalized, brain-based and clinical. Psychoanalysis never found a place in the academy, nor did romantic science. Freud (1993) Luria (1968; 2002) and Oliver Sacks' (1990; 1998) case studies read like literary fictions. It is no surprise that Freud won the Goethe prize.

The medical humanities—or today what is called the health humanities—attempt to put the human back into medicine. The health humanities are required in many medical schools across the country. Those who work in health humanities teach the study of memoir, autobiography and fiction—to medical students—in an attempt to humanize medicine.

Medical Anthropology

Arthur Frank, (1997) in the *The Wounded Storyteller,* suggests that *storytelling is* paramount to patient-centered medicine. Frank is a medical anthropologist who studies the human aspects of medical practice. Frank feels that the patient must have a say, a voice and a place in encounters with physicians. Otherwise, physicians can make medical mistakes because of cultural misunderstandings. Frank (1997) argues for a more holistic approach to medicine. Medical anthropologists study the phenomenology of patients' illness. Unlike other clinicians, medical anthropologists are consulted especially when there are cultural clashes with families that clinicians cannot resolve (e.g., Anne Fadiman's (2012) *The Spirit Catches You and You Fall Down*). Medical anthropologists and bioethicists work together to attempt to resolve family conflict with the medical staff, especially around end of life care.

I have written on Arthur Frank in detail elsewhere (Morris, 2008). However, I do want to highlight Frank's contributions as well as some of the problems I see with Franks' work. Briefly, what is relevant to this project are Frank's typologies. Frank (1997) argues that structural patterns across patients' stories emerge across cultures. Structures, patterns and typologies can be helpful, no doubt, when attempting to understand cultural conflict. But typologies—like any form of structuralism—can easily slide into over-simplifications.

Frank's (1997) narrative typologies basically fall into three types, or three narrative typologies: the first type he calls the "restitution narrative" (p. 77), the second, he calls the "quest narrative" (p. 115) and the third, he dubs the "chaos narrative" (p. 97). In other words, Frank argues that patients' narratives tend to fall into narrative patterns. As a chaplain, I have found Frank's narratives, on the one hand useful, but also problematic.

The "restitution narrative" (p. 77) is as follows: "Yesterday I was healthy, today I'm sick, but tomorrow I'll be healthy again" (p. 77). The "quest narrative" (Frank, 1997, p. 115) is as follows: "Illness is the occasion of a journey that becomes a quest. What is quested for may never be wholly clear, but the quest is defined by the ill person's belief that something is to be gained through the experience" (p. 115). The "chaos narrative" is as follows: "Chaos is opposite of restitution: its plot imagines life never getting better. Stories are chaotic in their absence of narrative order. Events are told... without sequence or discernible causality" (p. 97).

Especially with the emergence of covid-19, Frank's narrative typologies do not always capture the complexities of stories told from the patients' and/or families' perspectives. Of the three narratives Frank writes about, the one that I have heard most often—albeit, in much more complicated fashion—is the chaos narrative, or the narrative of *no narrative*. Sometimes I have heard all three types of narratives at once; at other times, patients' narratives do not fit into any of Frank's typologies.

Michel Foucault, in his final lectures the 1980s writes similarly about narrative structures found in ancient Greek philosophy. This is partly why, some consider Foucault to be a structuralist, not a poststructuralist. Most of Foucault's work is, indeed, structural in nature. For example, in book (1975)—in *Discipline and Punish*—Foucault (1975) writes about the similarities—or structure—across institutions such as prisons, mental institutions and schools. Briefly, Foucault argues that these various institutions—despite their obvious differences—all serve to discipline and punish.

Likewise, Foucault's (2011) *The Courage of Truth*, concerns character typologies found in ancient Greek philosophy. Foucault explores three kinds of character typologies common to ancient Greek philosophers who engage in what Foucault calls "truth-telling" (p. 15).

Foucault's (2011) three typologies of truth-tellers are: the "sage" (p. 16) the "prophet" (p. 15) and the "*parrhesiast*" (p. 19). For Foucault, the sage "lived in an essential withdrawal. He lived in silence" (p. 17). "He retired to the mountains" (p. 18). Foucault's "prophet" (p. 15) is the philosopher who allows the oracle to speak to him "in the form of a riddle" (p. 15). The oracle tells the philosopher what to think and what to do. Foucault's (2011) third type of philosopher he calls the "*parrhesiast*" (p. 18). This is the "truth-teller" who even risks death for the sake of the truth. Foucault, of course, is thinking of Socrates who risked death in order to be a "truth-teller." Risking death for the sake of the truth, Socrates exemplified what Foucault (2011) called the *courage of truth*.

Storytelling, Narrative and Typologies Upended

Typologies—like Frank's and Foucault's—do not always get played out in the real. There are no neat and tidy formulas for the ways in which storytellers tell their stories. Philosophers across time have demonstrated that they do not—in fact—fall into three typologies; the ancient Greek philosophers were much more complicated than that. The history of philosophy is about continual upheaval. Paradigm shifts occur because of disagreements. Paradigm shifts are the history of overturning ideas. Typologies suggest the lack up upheaval. Poststructuralists argue that structures are not cross cultural, that typologies are not similar across time and history. Storytelling—by patients—are never quite the same. And this is why the clinical case studies belie the differences between patients' stories. Unwittingly perhaps clinical case studies erase differences between patients, ignore cultural differences. This is why medical anthropologists and bioethicists have to be called in especially in cultural conflict with medical staff over end of life care. Cultures differ radically. And these cultural differences—sometimes come to a head when families get into heated arguments with physicians about end of life issues. Anne Fadiman (2012) documented this in the cultural collision of a Hmong family and physicians who did not understand the Hmong culture. The end result was catastrophe. Fadiman (2012) argued that if only a medical anthropologist would have been called in to mediate the case of the child who suffered from grand mal seizures which –in the end—caused irreversible brain damage, perhaps the end result of this story could have been otherwise. Fadiman called this child's case a cultural collision that ended badly. Fadiman's (2012) story is, in fact, tragic because the physicians did not understand the family's culture; if they had, perhaps the child would not have suffered so. Clinical case studies—that erase culture, race, class and gender—do not do justice to patients and their families. Medical chart notes that are seemingly clear cut and straight forward can—in the end—become highly problematic, especially when cultures clash.

Clinical case studies—especially—fail against what we are up against today, living through an unprecedented pandemic. Romantic science and medical anthropology—although both genres might be improvements over the sheer clinical—still cannot capture the complexities of a pandemic that is unprecedented. The medical community does not yet even have the language to describe what is happening, because we do not understand what is happening. This pandemic is beyond what it is we are able to think through; no form (whether clinical, romantic science or medical anthropology) can frame the stories of covid. Covid falls outside of representation and signification. Day after day, death after death, floor after floor the numbers keep going up. Covid patients are now spilling out into cardiac floors, the general hospital population. There are so many covid patients that there simply are not enough covid wards to isolate them. This could create a great danger to the general patient population because these floors are not isolation units.

Living in a world that has been upended by a pandemic demands a response like no other. Narrative typologies and sanitized chart notes do not help us understand the complexities of what we are facing. Further, the sanitization of covid as it is portrayed on TV—shields people from the truth of the ugliness of covid. Shielding people from the truth does not help them in the long run. And—perhaps more dangerously—shielding people from the truth plays into mythology that covid is not real.

Adorno (2008) remarks that "Bergson judged the non-conceptual to be the higher truth and sought it out in a stratum of more or less amorphous images residing beneath consciousness" (p. 70). The "non-conceptual," is the virus that is covid. This is an invisible enemy. One simply cannot conceptualize a virus—especially one that kills. Catastrophes like covid—cannot be reduced to concepts; catastrophes like covid cannot be contained by concepts. Covid as catastrophe is the intruder that invades the body in a way that belies. It is as Derrick Jensen (2000) might put it "a language older by far and deeper than words" (p. 2). Viruses are, indeed, far older than words. Adorno (2008) states that the idea "that there is a meaning despite everything—this seems to me more than we can reasonably expect anyone who has not been made stupid by philosophy [or I would add religion] to tolerate" (p. 19).

After witnessing countless, needless deaths, the idea that there is meaning in suffering seems nothing short of "stupid [ity]"—as Adorno puts it. To gloss over the horrors of meaningless deaths is nothing short of barbarism. Nothing makes sense anymore. Pandemics happen more often than we would like to believe. The Bubonic Plague in Europe is not the only pandemic that ever was. There were, in fact, many plagues in Europe which lasted years on end, only to return and then disappear and then return again.

There was another—less well known—epidemic tied to the flu in 1918, that has fallen out of historical narratives, perhaps because it is just too hard to think. Encephalitis lethargica occurred shortly after the 1918 flu epidemic—stealing the lives of untold numbers of people. Those who suffered from what was dubbed the sleeping sickness (or encephalitis lethargica) lived in comas for decades; they remained unconscious for the remainder of their lives. There was a brief period of time—however—where the drug L-Dopa did at first miraculously wake these patients up from their stupors. But L-Dopa backfired in the end and those who suffered with this horrid disease fell back into their comas or took on comatose behaviors.

Oliver Sacks (1990) intimated that there could have been a connection between the 1918 flu epidemic and encephalitis lethargica. Encephalitis lethargica is a complex disease, that is, in part, neurological. Sacks (1990) remarks that many "affected died in the acute stages of the sleeping-sickness, in states of coma so deep as to preclude arousal, or in states of sleeplessness so intense as to preclude sedation" (p. 13). Those who survived "would be conscious and aware—yet not fully awake; they would sit motionless and speechless all day in their chairs, totally lacking energy, impetus, initiative, motive, appetite, or desire".... They were ontologically dead" (p. 14). Sacks administered L-dopa to the victims of sleeping sickness at Mt. Carmel Hospital. Patients who miraculously woke up from this sleeping sickness—because of being treated with L-dopa—believed that they were still living some fifty years ago, as if no time had passed. However, the miracle did not last. L-dopa began to backfire. Patients began developing Parkinsonian-like symptoms, they developed spasticity problems, "myoclonic jerks... rigidity; desultory forceless movements." (p. 16). Some even became psychotic; others suffered a "wide range of tics" (p. 17). Encephalitis lethargica is the topic of Sacks' (1990) book *Awakenings*—which was subsequently made into a film.

Could there be a corollary between the covid 19 virus, the 1918 flu pandemic and encephalitis lethargica? Some neurologists worry. This possible connection between pandemics and subsequent neurological problems was first brought to my attention in discussion with a neurologist (name unknown) while working at the hospital. This neurologist, in fact, became alarmed when covid patients began to present with symptoms such as the inability to taste and smell. He stated that these symptoms are not benign. These are, in fact, neurological problems not to be taken lightly.

I found myself stunned when the neurologist made the connection between what happened after the 1918 flu epidemic, the onset of encephalitis lethargica, covid-19 and the inability to taste and smell. What is seemingly benign just might not be. What our future holds, no one can tell. The covid pandemic has morphed so many times and is so complicated that the medical community can barely keep up with variants, mutations and the massive numbers of deaths that continues to spiral out of control.

2

Speculative Fabulation and Unbearable Stories

Traditionally written historiography—sometimes referred to as history from above (e.g., military history, presidential history) is an example of what Walter Benjamin calls "homogeneous empty time" (2006a, p. 396). "Homogeneous empty time"—a complicated phrase echoing the writings of Henri Bergson—suggests that historiography—in its intersection with memory (relative to the concept of time)— obfuscates what history means in felt-time, in phenomenological time. That is, history as "homogeneous empty time" is as if time happens in a linear, orderly fashion. Time is, thus, emptied of its thickness, its complications, its intersections with space, fragmentation, gaps, and perspective. History as "homogeneous empty time"—is additive, calculated, if you will, and undergirds the status quo. Historiography, in this sense, is the story of winners, conquerors and colonists. Moreover, history as "homogeneous empty time" serves as a cover for the historian—who writes about the very history in which he may have participated in a crime. The historian might be guilty of being a "conspirator" (Benjamin, 2006b, p. 40) or collaborator.

As against "homogeneous empty time," Henri Bergson (2015) suggests that history is felt as "simultaneity" (p. 110) at the "intersection of time/ space" (p. 110). Historiography is felt as doubled. History *felt-as-memory*, that is, gets played out in parallel time(s), heterogeneous time(s).

It is crucial to note that Benjamin emphasizes that "history's original role as remembrance (*Eingedenken*).... marks history's final subjection to the modern concept of science" (2006a, p. 401). Modern science, in this context, means positivistic science. Historiography as positivism—historiography that gets folded into boxes, categories and methodologies that pretend toward objectivity—destroys not only personal memory but the very way in which that memory gets encoded into the historical archive.

Benjamin's (2006a) notion of "homogeneous empty time" echoes grand metanarratives with clear beginnings and endings. However, this is not the way history—especially in its intersection with memory—happens. Contrarily, Benjamin points out that "chronicles"—written as fragments or aphorisms—are more true to experience. Gregory Flaxman (2012)—in relation to this discussion—points out that according to Deleuze, Nietzsche's highly stylized aphorisms, or "fabulations" "as the very practice of philosophy" (p. xvi) hold "the power of invention" (p. xvi) by becoming "antagonistic to any image of thought" (p. xvi). Chronicles are, in a word, historical fabulations. Aphorisms are, in a word, poetic fabulations. Philosophy, in a word, is poetic fabulation, and indeed, what Donna Haraway (2011) might call "speculation fabulation" (p. 4).

Speculation: The Spy of Philosophy

Pragmatist philosopher Andrew Reck (1972) points out that "etymologically the term "speculation" has its origin in the Latin verb, *speculari,* meaning "to spy" (p. 10). Interestingly, spying was of interest to Walter Benjamin (2006a). Edgar Allan Poe, who fascinated Benjamin, wrote detective stories. Most think of Poe as the master of horror stories. However, Poe also wrote detective stories, as he was interested in the figure of the spy. To spy means to engage in speculation.

Michel Foucault (2011) points out that the Greek philosopher "Epictetus explains that the Cynic's role is to exercise the office of the spy... sent ahead of the army to observe as unobtrusively as possible what the enemy is doing" (p. 167). The Cynic-as-spy "will return to announce the truth" (Foucault, 2011, p. 167). Foucault (2011) explains: "The Cynic is the man with the staff, the beggar's pouch, the cloak, the man in sandals or bare feet, the man with the long beard, the dirty man. He is also the man who roams, who is not integrated into society" (p. 170). The Cynic, therefore, engaged in a philosophy of spying.

Speculation—broadly speaking—intersects with economics, law, literary fiction and philosophy. One of the oldest meanings of speculation—in the history of Western philosophy—is wonder. Philosophy, it is said, begins with wonder. Or, perhaps philosophy begins with doubt, as in the case of Descartes. Either way, wonder and doubt are both forms of speculation.

In *The Nichomachean Ethics* (1987) Aristotle claims that a "prominent" life includes the "sensual" the "political" and the "speculative" (p. 15). Aristotle weaves these various ideas—hither and yon—leaving the reader perplexed. The reader is led to believe—throughout the body of the text—that *living* right (*eudamonia*) meant *doing* right. That is, good deeds in the realm of the political—for Aristotle—seemed to win out over contemplation. But by Book X in *The Ethics*, Aristotle will come back around to Plato's position that contemplation—or speculation—wins the day, over against doing, or action.

In Book II of *The Ethics*, Aristotle writes that courageous or noble characters are best exemplified by courageous or noble deeds. Further, pontificating about virtue was not enough: one had to *engage* in virtuous deeds. Aristotle (1987) claims: "Our present study is not, like other studies, purely speculative in its intention; for the object of our enquiry is not to know the nature of virtue but to become ourselves virtuous" (p. 44). However, Aristotle contradicts himself later on, as I said previously.

Aristotle continues to hedge between action and speculation in the opening of Book II. Here, Aristotle sets "intellectual virtue" over against "moral virtue" (p. 42)—seemingly driving a wedge between speculation and action. Aristotle drives home this point by stating that "intellectual virtue is both originated and fostered mainly by teaching" (p. 43), while "moral virtue… is the outcome of habit, and… is derived by a slight deflexion [spelling in the original] from habit" (p. 43). Aristotle intimates that "intellectual" virtue reigns supreme. Moral virtue is born out of bad habits; to rely on habit is to live badly.

Conversely, "Intellectual virtue"—because one acquires it through "teaching" "foster[s]" (p. 43) the speculative. Socrates—in contradistinction to Aristotle—argued that he never actually taught anyone anything. Rather—drawing on Plato's theory of recollection—Socrates said that he was a midwife helping others to recall what they already knew but simply forgot.

Educare, the Latin root of the word education, similarly means to draw out. Teaching is not a matter of didactics. In fact, it is just the opposite. Teaching is the art of opening spaces for others to find their own way, to discover—with some guidance perhaps—what knowledges are most worthwhile to them. Teachers create the conditions for students to explore what is most meaningful to them.

When Socrates was put on trial in Plato's (2008) *Apology* for corrupting the youth, his defense was that he was not guilty of any crime because he never taught anyone anything; therefore he could not have corrupted the youth because he taught them nothing. Socrates helped others to recover what he believed to be forgotten knowledge. Plato, it must be noted, felt that contemplation or speculation won out over against action and the life of the sensuous, or the life of the senses. In fact, Plato kicked the poets out of the Republic because he felt that poetry was little more than an expression of sensuous life. On this, I think Plato took a wrong turn, for poetry is the highest form of language; poetry and philosophy split with Plato, and that is where philosophy, I think, began to move in the wrong direction. What else is philosophy but a form of poetics?

Aristotle (1996)—although he seemed more sympathetic to the work of the poets and in fact wrote a book called the *Poetics*—came back round to Plato's position at the end of the day. Like Plato, Aristotle claimed that speculation ultimately won out. In fact, in Book X of *The Ethics* Aristotle claims that "contemplation" (p. 343) or "speculation" (p. 343) is the path toward *Eudamonia*. Aristotle argues that "speculation is the highest activity" (p. 343). Aristotle suggests that it is "degrad[ing] (p. 348)" to think that the Gods engage in any kind of "moral action" (p. 348). "We may go through the whole category of virtues, and it will appear that whatever relates to moral action is petty and unworthy of the Gods" (p. 348). Mortals must mirror the Gods who honor speculation.

Aristotle—as was mentioned at the outset of this chapter—famously states that philosophy begins in wonder. But isn't wonder more than speculation? Doesn't wonder include intuition, perception, reverie and dreams? Gaston Bachelard thought so. But of course, Bachelard was so entirely different from Aristotle that perhaps that comparison is not a good one. However, Aristotle did not rule out intuition as being important to building character. And Socrates did not discount the possibility of death being akin to dreaming. If philosophy beings in wonder and ends in speculation—as Aristotle puts it—how is wonder akin to speculation? Or is wonder—in actuality—a form of speculation?

Alice in Wonderland—by Lewis Carol—is at once wonder, fantasy, fable and political satire. Wonderment is also that which cannot be known. Andrew Reck (1972) points out that for A.N. Whitehead speculation (like wonder?) implied "a disturbing element" (p. 2): "[T]he flight after the unattainable" (cited in Reck, p. 2). Here, speculation is a disturbance of sorts. Speculation is a "flight" after what cannot be known. The Greek myth of Icarus captures that "disturbing" nature of the "flight of the unattainable." Isn't wonder also a "flight of the unattainable?"

David Lemming (2014) tells the story of Icarus: this is the "flight of the unattainable" which does not end well. Dadedalus, the wing-maker, if you will, warned Icarus:

> Icarus, I advise you to take a middle course. If you fly too low, the sea will soak the wings; if you fly too high, the sun's heat will burn them. Fly between the sea and sun! (cited in Lemming, 2014, p. 303)

Dadedalus'–middle way, like Aristotle's mean—suggests that engaging in excess does not end well. This myth, or fable, which is the root of the word fabulation, is a cautionary tale. The ending of this fable reads thusly:

> [D]rawn by a desire to reach the heavens, took his course too high. The burning heat of the nearby sun softened the scented wax that fastened the wings. The wax melted: Icarus moved his arms, now uncovered, and without the wings to drive him on, vainly beat the air. Even as he called upon his father's name the sea received him and from him took his name. (cited in Lemming, 2014, p. 304)

Icarus took the "flight of the unattainable" (cited in Reck, 1972, p. 2). But in this case, the end result was catastrophe. Despite the possibility of bad endings, "flights of the unattainable," Andrew Reck (1972) argues, can offer us an "astonishing vision" (p. 3).

The film by Julian Schnabel (2018)—*At Eternity's Gate*—about van Gough depicts the life of an artist who engages in "astonishing vision" (Reck, 1972, p. 3). Van Gough delved deeply into philosophical questions about the meaning of life and death. Painting raised these kinds of questions for Van Gough. Painting, like poetry, raises profound issues, albeit in a preverbal way. Questions of life and death—no matter how they come about—are, indeed, speculative. A priest in a mental asylum in which Van Gough is interned—acts as an interrogator. The priest—who doubts Van Gough's sanity, asks: how do you *know* you are a painter? Van Gough's reply to the priest was this: I know I am a painter because I am, because God made me a painter. I am what I am, Van Gough replies. Van Gough's "desire to reach the heavens" like Icarus (in Lemming, 2014, p. 304) allowed him to let his imagination take flight. To take flight—in art, in poetry, in painting or philosophy, means risk-taking. Speculation is a form of risk-taking. To speculate is to guess, to wonder, to imagine.

Speculation birthed—what Andrew Reck (1972) considers to be—"all the great philosophers from Thales to Whitehead" (p. 2). In fact, Reck insists that speculative philosophy is, indeed, *"metaphysical"* (italics in the original, p. 2). I ask what philosophy is not speculative? What philosophy—at bottom is not—metaphysical? Questions of life and death, being and becoming, reason and intuition, time and space, the one and the many—are all metaphysical quandaries. Perhaps logic—in its most narrow definition—is not metaphysical. But one could argue that late Wittgenstein (1958) engaged in metaphysics. Questions of theology (e.g., Kierkegaard (1983) and Royce (2001)), questions of cosmology (e.g., A.N. Whitehead (1927) and Democritus' (2010)) questions of time (Henri Bergson (2015) and Martin Heidegger (1962)) are all metaphysical and speculative. Imagine philosophy devoid of this richness? What would be left without metaphysical speculation?

Wittgenstein (1922) once argued in the *Tractatus*—that if a problem of philosophy cannot be demonstrated through logic, it is not a philosophical problem. But Wittgenstein later stated that he was wrong. As Wittgenstein (1958) matured as a philosopher, his work became more aphoristic and puzzling, indeed, metaphysical and speculative.

Speculative fabulation is sometimes associated with science fiction. However, Donna Haraway (2011) broadens the meaning of speculative fabulation in her essay *SF: Speculative Fabulation and String Figures*. Haraway (2011) focuses on the term "fabulation," but does not drive a wedge between the speculative and fabulation; in fact, she collapses these terms. Haraway (2011) states that fabulation is a "fictional multiple integral equation" (p. 4) as both "flawed trope" (p. 4) and "serious joke" (p. 4). She goes on to map out a seemingly absurd and fictional mathematical equation that serves as a satire of mathematics and science. Haraway points out that both mathematics and science are fabulations of sorts.

Haraway (2011)—focusing on fabulation—emphasizes collapsing dualisms. Haraway (2011) states "code alteration mutates things" (p. 7). Mutations, i.e. viruses, are far more complicated than variants adding or subtracting this or that genomic sequence. Haraway (2011), in the spirit of multiplicity, says that the way in which viruses mutate are multiples. Time is also multiple. She states that time(s) are "multi-scaluar... entangled" (p. 4).

For Haraway (2011), "storytelling" contains "multispecies worlding in SF modes" (p. 5). Here, Haraway refers to Navajo "string figures" meaning "coyotes running opposite ways" (np). String-figure games might seem like child's play, but, in fact, Haraway uses string-figures as metaphors for theoretical physics, biopolitics, "biogeochemistry" and more. Haraway attempts to collapse quantum physics, biopolitics, time(s), space(s), ecosphere(s). Haraway (2011) states that *"Homo Sapiens"* "think they know what a line is" (p. 5). Does this sentence not sum up Wittgenstein's (1922) *Tractatus*? Recall, Wittgenstein argues that if logic cannot demonstrate a problem, then it is not a problem of philosophy. Philosophers took the *Tractatus* as the gospel of philosophy, as Andrew Reck (1972) points out, denigrating metaphysics. And still today, it is evident—especially in the Oxbridge tradition—that analytic philosophy has eclipsed metaphysics. Yet, one might argue that logic is but a game. And yet, it is a dangerous game. Today, as I see it, the end result of logic is AI. Zizek (2020) warns that AI is veering into dangerous territory, for AI can read people's thoughts. Some suggest that AI has the capacity to control peoples' thoughts as well.

Andrew Reck (1972) cites his mentor at Yale, Paul Weiss who wrote eloquently about what it means to think (to speculate). Risk-taking is part of the web and woof of intellectual life as scholars who

> Should display "humility in the attitude... freedom from provincialism... catholicity of spirit, some courage too," and while they [intellectuals] rely upon "the insight and wisdom of others," they should never merely repeat what has already been said. (p. 5).

And still, university culture encourages "provincialism" the lack of "catholicity of spirit" the lack of "courage." Little has changed since 1950 as university culture is not a place that encourages risk, inventiveness, flying too close to the sun. Invention and creativity are, in fact, discouraged. Mediocrity is the key to survival in the university. Nobel Prize–winning scientist Sydney Brenner (2014) argues that the problem with academic journals and the peer review process is it is "very distorted" and "completely corrupt." The peer review process results, Brenner (2014) argues, in "a regression to the mean" (np, retractionwatch.com). Scholarship that is too experimental or that is not understood by reviewers, although it could be groundbreaking and quite important, mostly gets rejected. Who decides what gets published and what does not is a highly political question. And in this case, the golden mean—Aristotle's mantra—is detrimental to academic fields. If reviewers cannot understand what it is that they are reviewing and toss out important scholarship, what they are actually doing is perpetuating the status quo. And this is what "provincialism" in academe is.

Chronicles as Speculative Fabulation

A Berlin Chronicle is a short story Walter Benjamin (1978) wrote about growing up in Berlin. Writing about childhood is a kind of fabulation. No one can remember their childhoods as they actually happened. Freud reminds that getting at the truth of childhood is not what matters. Rather, what is more important is what we do with the memories that we have—whether they are true or not. Ironically, what might be more important when writing a chronicle of childhood—like Benjamin's—is what gets left out, or forgotten. In any event, whether we think we remember events as they happened, or whether we forgot what happened, both remembering and forgetting are forms of fabulation.

Memories of childhood are not recalled in a linear, chronological fashion. A chronicle of childhood is a patchwork or fragmented compilation of mixed-up memories and blank spots. Perhaps we fill in those blank spots with things that never existed. Memories hides in half-forgotten days.

Benjamin states that traditional forms of historiography are little more than glosses over "melancholy" (2016, p. 16) as well as glosses over the ontological experience of living in a continual "state of horror" (2016, p, 16). Like historiography, then, one might surmise—and Freud would concur—that childhood chronicles, or memoirs can serve to either "gloss over" "states of horror" or not. D.W. Winnicott asked throughout his work: to what use do we put our memories? Freud asked the same question. What do we do with the memories of childhood—or fabulations, if you will—that we have? To what use do we put the gaps in our memories, the blank spaces, the forgetting?

Homogeneous Empty Time

Objective historical methodologies create, in part, the problem of getting stuck in a loop of "homogeneous empty time," as Benjamin (2006a) puts it. History is not linear, chronological, additive. But because of the stultification of historical methodologies, historiography seems as if its narrative is, in fact, linear, chronological and additive. History is anything but homogeneous. The witting or unwitting erasure of history occurs through historians' "objective" methodology, especially around unpalatable events, or what Holocaust historians term unusable pasts.

In Benjamin's (2006a) *Theses on the Philosophy of History* "homogeneous empty time" gets upended by his Messianic notion of history as felt-time. History unfolds in an almost mystical sense. Memory and history are intertwined for Benjamin, whereas most historians drive a wedge between these concepts. For Benjamin, memories "flash" up in sudden illuminations. "Images" (2006a, p. 391), Benjamin points out—are experienced as "bursts" or "flashes" (2006a, p. 390). Benjamin is one of the few philosophers in the Western tradition—besides Derrida—who embraces Messianism. Ironically, in the Jewish tradition the Messianic is more about memory work than about anticipating the future. Although Elijah—the prophet—is to-come, the work in the now-time, as Benjamin might have put it, and the remembrance of those who have come before us, is more important than anticipating the future. Perhaps this is why

Benjamin was fascinated by Paul Klee's *Angelus Novus*, the painting of the angel with his wings stuck, being blown backwards. Benjamin's Philosophy of History is perhaps the most unusual in the history of philosophy because it is both a kind of mysticism and a kind of speculation on memory. Hegel's philosophy of history is completely counter to Benjamin's in that it is about the future; but there is nothing human about Hegel's history of philosophy, for Spirit sweeps everything in its way into the future. Benjamin's philosophy of history is human. It is a work of mourning; it concerns the very stuff of suffering—the most human of emotions.

Positivistic historiography is little more than a "procedure that is additive: it musters a mass of data to fill the homogeneous empty time" (p. 360). Data-driven historiography serves to normalize and perpetuate the status quo. In fact, historians can be complicit in what Hannah Arendt (2006) calls the banality of evil. Adorno (2005) put it this way: "Normality is death" (p. 56). "Homogeneous empty time" (Benjamin, 2006a) is also death. Benjamin (2006a) states that history is a "piling up" of disasters.

But revisionist historians—like Holocaust deniers—want to erase the "piling up" of disasters by pretending that the Holocaust did not occur; or revisionists re-write—or even unwrite the past to make it more palatable. But erasing disastrous histories is in itself disastrous. Benjamin (2006a) argues that "the fight for the oppressed past" (p. 396) is our responsibility. Thus, Benjamin (2006a) calls for a "theoretical armature" (p. 396) that is able to protect the past from its own erasure. History cannot speak for itself: it must be archived, theorized, opening spaces that allow for critique and condemnation of normalization, forgetfulness and erasure.

Trauma

History is the piling up of horrors, Benjamin says. It is also the piling up of pandemics, plagues. Covid-19 is indeed a plague, a pandemic. There have been many pandemics in history and more are to come. But what we are living through is unprecedented; most of us did not live through the 1918 flu pandemic. Even if we did, the two pandemics are not the same; they are not homogenous.

In the context of the covid-19 pandemic it is imperative to "fight for the oppressed past" (Benjamin, 2006a, p. 396). We are already beginning to see that this pandemic is being unwritten or rewritten and glossed over by those who claim it is not real, or that it is just like the flu, or that it is not dangerous. It seems unthinkable that covid has gotten politicized and turned into something that it is not. The truth is right in front of us. And yet those reactionary voices of utter denial—that covid is not real—speak loudly and wield power. Republican led states are now suffering the fallout of reactionary governing, as the elderly, children and young adults are not only getting sick, but are dying in increasing numbers. Some seem completely ignorant of history and eschew science altogether in the name of liberty and freedom. Oliver Sacks (1990) cites H.L. Mencken as he recalls the erasure of the 1918 flu epidemic; both the flu pandemic and encephalitis lethargica have strangely been absent from our history books. Mencken remarked that

> The epidemic is seldom mentioned, and most Americans have apparently forgotten it. This is not surprising. The human mind always tries to expunge the intolerable from memory, just as it tries to conceal it while current. (Mencken, cited in Sacks, p. 13)

Some historians suggest that one of the reasons Americans do not recall the 1918 flu pandemic is because people died so quickly that they did not have time to write about or record what had happened to them. The 1918 flu pandemic was overshadowed by WW1. This erasure was compounded by the fact that President Wilson lied about the flu pandemic and censored the press. But soldiers were dying more from the flu than from combat on the battlefield.

Benjamin (2006a) states that the "angel of history"—drawing on Paul Klee's painting *Angelus Novaus*—whose wings are stuck open and "blown" backwards by the "storm" of "progress" (p. 392), illuminates how we are traveling backwards—despite the development of vaccines—as the storm of covid is killing so many. The "storm" of covid "keeps piling wreckage upon wreckage" (p. 392). This "wreckage upon wreckage" must not be rewritten as a more palatable or usable past.

The Life Never Lived

Psychoanalyst Adam Phillips (2012) writes that what we tend to ignore has more importance than what we pay attention to. Phillips claims that fantasies—that we ignore—about the life never lived might actually be more important than the life that we are actually living. Phillips asks: "How much of our so-called mental life is about the lives we are not living, the lives we are missing out on, the lives we could be leading but for some reason are not" (p. xi). Interestingly Walter

Benjamin (2016) addresses this issue as well, albeit in a different manner. He asks us to think about

> *Then path that you wanted to take*
> *The letter you wanted to write*
> *The man that you wanted to rescue*
> *The seat that you wanted to occupy*
> *The woman that you wanted to follow*
> *The word that you wanted to hear*
> (italics in the original, p. 27)

Why did we not take the path we really wanted to take? These questions become more pronounced if we experience serious illness.

Covid-19 has forced many to re-evaluate their lives. Sequestered at home, sheltering in place for months on end, feeling closed-in and isolated, second thoughts occur about a life never lived, a life one wanted to live but never did. Reflection and regret emerge when one is forced to sit still and think. "If not now, when?" asked Hillel the Elder, the ancient Talmudist. There is a kind of mourning that accompanies a life that was never lived. To speculate about what if or if I had just done X brings with it certain melancholia.

Speculation, as it is usually discussed in philosophy, lacks the psychological aspect of mourning and melancholia—especially when one wonders what if, why didn't I do X, or perhaps I could have done something differently with my life. To think that one's life could have been otherwise and wish that it could have been otherwise—-what Henry James might have called the *figure in the carpet*—leads to obsessive thoughts, depression, anguish. There comes a time in one's life when it is too late to do the things we always wanted to do. As we age, these thoughts become more pronounced. The colleges we never attended, the degrees we never got, the careers that never worked out—*figures in the carpet* of lives not lived. We tell ourselves stories about the lives we never lived; mourning and melancholia are not simply concepts, they are real lived anguishes. The regret over the book never written or the last conversation we could have had with our parents before they died—linger in memory. "Flights after the unattainable" (Reck, 1972, p. 2) sometimes fill us with grief, not wonder, especially if we miss the mark and fail. Failures of lives never lived haunt. It is curious that philosophers rarely address the psychological aspects of speculation.

Psychoanalysis—in concert with philosophy—adds a certain richness that philosophy lacks. While philosophy has things to offer, so too does psychoanalysis. But these two disciplines—as Jean-Luc Nancy and Avital Ronell might suggest—go hand-in-glove. One cannot separate the psychic life from the philosophical life, but psyche got left out of the history of philosophy. This is curious because Socrates' final words to his disciples concerned psyche, or the soul. He said to them: take care of yourselves. Care of the soul, a phrase later taken up by Foucault, Jungian analysts such as James Hillman and Thomas Moore, is a crucial aspect of Socrates' work. But care of the soul tends to get overshadowed by Plato's theory of recollection or his work on The Republic. The soul fell away as a concept even in psychology, as it became medicalized in the late 19th century. But the root of the word psychology—psyche—means soul. Psychoanalytically-informed chaplaincy draws on the notion of the soul but because chaplaincy, too, has become more medicalized and standardized, soul has fallen away from that discipline as well. The soul—a term associated mostly with theology—has lost its way. Some philosophers feel that this word is too theological; some theologians are uncomfortable with this word because it cannot be systematized. Empiricism—which is based on materiality—has little truck with soul. But it seems to me that this notion is an important one that needs resuscitation.

The soul is a mystical term; it cannot be categorized or systematized. The soul is not based in the materiality of the brain; the soul is not the same thing as the mind. Let me be clear, however. I am not arguing for an evangelical notion of the soul, that the soul is more important than the body or life itself. The soul is embodied and it is part and parcel of speculation, perception, mourning and melancholia. The soul is a concept that cannot be conceptualized; perhaps it is a non-concept. The soul is that ineffable something that lends to a kind of depth of thought and emotion. Speculative fabulation is a kind of soul-work as well. There is nothing trivial about speculative fabulation. When one constructs stories—even if they lack narrative structure—in the midst of catastrophe, the soul lends depth to those stories. The stories that I draw on later in the book, say by Terry Tempest Williams and Joan Didion, are indeed soulful: stories without depth—without soul—reside in the world of unthought language and jargon. Jargon and everyday language cannot capture soulful storytelling. And this, I think, is one of the main problems with academic writing, especially the writing found in academic journals. Many articles in academic journals are jargon-filled and soulless. Academics are encouraged to write in a scientistic style. William James was excoriated for his philosophical style, his embellished language; Lucretius—the ancient poet—has been forgotten by most philosophers or is left out of the philosophical canon altogether because of the long-standing rift between poetry and philosophy. The soul is a poetic concept; it is a metaphor.

During the pandemic—when the chaplain is called in—the patient is nearing death. The chaplain is not a scientist, not a physician. The chaplain is not a priest. The chaplain is the one who holds the stories of the Other; a soulless chaplain should not be a chaplain. Care of the soul is the heart of the profession of chaplaincy. Ironically, soul-work in chaplaincy is carried out mostly in silence and meditation. This is something that Thomas Merton—the trappist monk to whom I dedicate an entire chapter in this book—understood well. Trappist monks take a vow of silence. Merton felt that silence is the heart of the soul; the divine is found not in idle chatter or spouting biblical passages, but in silent meditation on the deeply theological, the deeply philosophical questions of life and death.

Perception and the Body

Maurice Merleau-Ponty (1989) opens up spaces to think in a more embodied way about historiography, storytelling, biography and autobiography in the context of covid-19. In *The Primacy of Perception* Merleau-Ponty (1989) states: "History is other people; it is interrelationships" (p. 25). Merleau-Ponty (2010) makes few references to history in his major work, *Phenomenology of Perception*. However, early on—in the preface—he does state that "intersubjectivity" (2010, p. xxii, xiv) is located "in a historical situation" (xiv). Merleau-Ponty put the body in the midst of the world, in fact; he remarked that "the body has its world" (2010, p. 162). There is no split between the body and the world. The body is the world as the world is the body. This being-in-the-world is felt phenomenologically as an immersion. Merleau-Ponty mentions that as painters look at objects, the objects look back at painters.

While Kant (2007) claims that space and time are structures in the mind, Merleau-Ponty (2010) claims that the body "inhabit[s] space and time" (p. 161). Merleau-Ponty (2010) emphasizes: "I am not in space and time, nor do I conceive space and time [which is Kant's position]; I belong to them, my body combines with them and includes them" (p. 161). Kant (2007) does not do much, if anything with the concept of the body.

Perhaps Benjamin's Messianic time is felt as an *out of body* experience, but still, one needs a body to have an out of body experience to begin with. The other important idea of Messianic time is that it is something that is perceived, perhaps mysteriously. Messianic time is, after all, a perception. Merleau-Ponty (1989) grounds the body, thought and experience, history and interrelations in perception. But again, this is not a disembodied perception: it is an embodied perception. And it is this emphasis on embodiment-in-the-midst-of-the-world that makes Merleau-Ponty different from many other philosophers who preceded him.

Merleau-Ponty (2010) states that "experience breaks forth into things" (p. 353). Merleau-Ponty (2010)—in a Freudian moment—states that "Every sensation carries with it the germ of a dream" (p. 250). For Merleau-Ponty (2010) the dream is not transcendent, ascending in a fashion akin to the biblical Jacob, who climbs a ladder. Merleau-Ponty (2010) also remarks that the sky is not transcendent either. He claims: "I am not set over against it[the sky] as an acosmic subject; I do not possess it in thought... I abandon myself to it and plunge into the mystery, it 'thinks itself within me.' I am the sky itself" (p. 249). Merleau-Ponty's position is akin to ecologist Terry Tempest Williams (2001) who says, "I am desert. I am mountains. I am Great Salt Lake" (p. 29). Like Williams, Merleau-Ponty (2010) claims that the body is not separate and distinct from the world, the body is the world and the world is the body.

Perception is not clear: Ludwig Wittgenstein's Perception as a Curious Puzzle

Wittgenstein (1958) suggests in the *Philosophical Investigations* that perception is like a "puzzle" and in fact, perception is rather puzzling. In other words, to perceive is akin to a "puzzle-picture" (p. 196e). Further, one becomes puzzled while trying to figure out what one is perceiving in that picture. Drawing on *Facts and Fable in Psychology*—by one Jastrow (cited in Wittgenstein, 1958)—Wittgenstein reproduces a "puzzle-picture" (196e) of a "duck-rabbit" (p. 194e, 1958). If one perceives the duck-rabbit one way (as a duck) it is impossible to simultaneously see the rabbit. If one perceives the duck-rabbit as a duck—on first look—it is very difficult, if not impossible, to see the rabbit. Depending upon one's perception, the picture *puzzles* because it is difficult to see two differing perceptions simultaneously. On a second look, one must shift one's perception—consciously—to see something other than what one saw the first time round. Now, this is a curious phenomenon. These kinds of perceptual problems happen all the time in real life but most ignore this puzzling occurrence, making little of it. But Wittgenstein shows why it is that one might think more seriously about perceptual puzzles that occur rather frequently in life. One might wonder why this kind of experience is not given much thought. Recall, Adam Phillips (2012) stresses that what we ignore—in this case altered perceptions—is more important than what we pay attention to.

Wittgenstein (1958) comments on another kind of perceptual puzzle: "I must distinguish between the 'continuous seeing' of an aspect and the 'dawning' of an aspect"(p. 194e). How is it that something suddenly changes right in front of one's eyes? What is it that makes perception shift? That is the puzzle at hand. Is there a clear answer for this shift? No. And that is the mystery of perception. Perception, for Wittgenstein, is a game of illusions.

Shifting perceptions in the picture-puzzle of the duck-rabbit and the altered state of perception in what Wittgenstein calls "the dawning of an aspect" are questions about the *mystery* of perception. What exactly is the "dawning of an aspect"? Wittgenstein wonders (1958, p. 194e). When perception mysteriously shifts, a new "aspect" "dawns." Is this not akin to fabulation? A game of illusions? Interestingly Wittgenstein (1958) repeats the word game when talking about language having family resemblances. When Wittgenstein comments on "language-games" he compares them to "board-games, card-games, ball-games" (p. 31e). Is not the duck-rabbit "puzzle-picture" a game of illusions?

Perception is partly a game of fabulation; it is a mystery that the mind plays tricks on itself. It is notable that perception—as a serious philosophical subject— has been taken up by just a few 20th-century philosophers in the Western tradition (see, for example, Merleau-Ponty, 2010; Jean-Luc Nancy, 1996; Jacques Derrida, 2005; Wittgenstein, 1958). Perception as a puzzle, as Wittgenstein (1958) points out, is rather puzzling. Interestingly, Wittgenstein (1958) calls the duck-rabbit a puzzle-picture, not a picture-puzzle. The meaning of a puzzle-picture is not the same as a picture-puzzle. In effect, the "language-game" of switching the words picture and puzzle makes a difference perceptually. This is another example of how perception shifts through a linguistic sleight-of-hand.

Wittgenstein (1958) remarks that shifts in perception, shifts in language-games, are "elastic" (p. 198e) and imbued with "ambiguity" (195e). Perception can also shift the way one sees another person. All of a sudden a person looks differently. Wittgenstein gives the example of not recognizing someone and then suddenly recognizing him. How is it that a face can seemingly change? Wittgenstein (1958) states: "I meet someone whom I have not seen for years; I see him clearly, but fail to know him. Suddenly I know him, I see the old face in the altered one" (p. 197e). This "flashing of an aspect" (p. 197e) is partly "visual" and partly "thought" (p. 197e).

Oliver Sacks, a neurologist, reported that he suffered from a condition in which he could not recognize the faces of people he knew—at all. He would come back from his appointment with his psychiatrist, he tells us, run into him in an elevator, and not recognize him at all. Sacks stated that he suffered from what is called *prosopagnosia,* a neurological problem. One must then ask the question whether neurology is, in some way, related to perception? Even if it is, shifts in perception cannot be fully explained. The mystery of perception remains.

Perhaps *prosopagnosia* is radically different from a perceptual shift in the duck-rabbit puzzle-picture. Still, it is important to note that the very ability to perceive anything at all can be inhibited by neurological diseases. Neurologists might be able to use medical terminology to describe a disturbance in mental functioning, but there is more to the mind than its materiality.

Perception as it is related to fable, fabulation and speculation, or speculative fabulation does not mean twisting the truth into non-truth. Storytelling as speculative fabulation is not non-truth, nor is it post-truth, revisionism or lies. In the context of unbearable stories of covid and the archivization of this pandemic, yes speculation comes into play. We can only speculate what is happening at this historical juncture, for time slips as the process of archivization takes place. The puzzle of perception comes into play as well in the context of this pandemic. It is very difficult to perceive what is right in front of us as historicity is ever-moving; capturing the moving object of historicity is indeed puzzling and is a puzzle in and of itself. The pieces of the puzzle are forever changing right in front of us, right before our eyes. As the pandemic changes, as the variants continue to mutate, our perception of the pandemic changes as well. One day the media reports that the pandemic is soon coming to an end; the next day a new variant pops up and the pandemic starts all over again, but worse. This seems a never-ending puzzle for scientists. One day they say that the vaccines are efficacious. The next day, they qualify this by saying that the vaccines are efficacious up to a point. Breakthrough cases even of the fully vaccinated are not uncommon. The next variant on the horizon, some suggest, might be able to outwit the vaccines altogether. New vaccines are on the horizon. The news reports that the next pandemic after covid will be even worse. We do not know what that will be, the bird-flu? But when. How do we psychologically manage all of this jumbled data. As covid numbers go up in one part of the country, they go down in another; as the covid numbers devastate some nations around the globe; other nations are seeing the numbers and deaths go down. We are living in a topsy-turvy world.

Speculative fabulation is a complicated concept to grasp as it applies to this pandemic. To fabulate, again, in this case, is not to make up lies. Stories are fabulations—or social constructions. Social constructions are not lies. To speculate and to engage in storytelling are highly complex psychological and philosophical activities. Perception also comes into play. How we perceive what is right in front of us, how we speculate what is right in front of us, is perhaps the most difficult task at hand. It is nearly impossible to see—or to perceive—what is right in front of us. This pandemic is, indeed, right in front of us, and we cannot see it or perceive it in any clear manner. As the pandemic changes so do our perceptions of it.

Speculation—as it has been traditionally perceived in the history of Western philosophy as contemplation, or rationality—might not make much sense against what it is we are living through. Although we might have time to become contemplative—if we are in quarantine, or if we get sick from covid—this kind of contemplation is not the same, say, as what it is that philosophers do. In fact, too much time in isolation turns contemplation into a kind of torment. Dwelling on what is happening during this pandemic can lead to obsessing over the horror, thoughts take on their own thoughts and those thoughts might lead to psychological melt-down. Speculation, as it was conceived by Aristotle or Plato, for example, was the highest form of intellectual activity. The senses, perception, action or doing was thought to only get in the way of speculation, or be secondary to the process of speculation. But do we not speculate, perceive, act and sense simultaneously? Haraway's move to "implode" concepts is useful here because one comes to understand—especially during lockdown and isolation—that thought and perception, action and non-action, the conceptual and non-conceptual, emotions and sensations all happen simultaneously. Speculation is not detachment from the body; speculation is embodied, sensed, felt, lived and so forth. Speculative fabulation—when thinking about our own stories during covid—is always already opened to change, alteration; speculative fabulation, indeed, is a process, it is in process, it is not static or stable. Memories, nightmares, depression, transference, denial are all part of speculative fabulation—for thinking is not merely intellectual, it is also deeply psychological and moreover, much of the stories we tell ourselves are driven by the unconscious. There is a mystery about storytelling; narrative is not always narrative: chronicles are fragmented, broken up, and mixed up. Thought is shot through with fantasy, fabulation, perception and unsolvable puzzles.

In the context of covid-19, speculative fabulation differs from the way this phrase has been used in science fiction, for example. Speculative fabulation is a kind of mourning work, in the way that I would like to re-frame and reconceptualize this phrase. Although this chapter began in wonder and in a discussion of Aristotle, this chapter ends in mourning. The pandemic we are living through is difficult to conceptualize for many reasons but most of all, as we are in the midst of this chaos and sadness, mourning can become overwhelming. Stories about suffering—in the context of this pandemic—and that which we speculate about are steeped in mourning, melancholia and remembrance. Thus, speculative fabulation must be a kind of memory work, a kind of soul-work—in this context. Mourning, melancholia and memory work puzzle. Perceptions change because perceptions are shot through with emotion, with the what-ifs, or could I have done something differently. Facing mortality, witnessing the death of the Other, changes one's perception, the way in which one thinks about the past and what is to come.

3

Jacques Derrida's Concepts: Metaphors for Unbearable Stories

In order to understand Derrida, we must first begin with some key ideas found in the work of Emmanuel Levinas. I argue that Levinas sets the stage for Derrida. In fact, Derrida is deeply indebted to Levinas, especially around the concept of alterity—-especially as this relates to Derrida's unwieldy notions of the archive, the trace and differance. These unwieldy concepts can help us think through the current crisis of covid-19.

Emmanuel Levinas (1985) argues that one's "authentic relationship" to "the other" concerns ethicality; relationships to the Other demand "response or responsibility" (p. 88). Levinas notably writes about the metaphor of the "face" of the Other. The face is not a literal term; the face is a metaphor, it is not something visual, something that one sees. The face is, rather, a signifier for God. God is the face of the Other. Therefore, the moral imperative against killing has directly to do with the Face of the Other—that is God. In other words, thou shalt not kill the Other because the Other is the face of God. Levinas (1985) declares that "[i]n the access to the face there is certainly an access to the idea of God" (p. 92). The ethicality not to kill the Other means killing the Other is the equivalent of killing God. Levinas (1996) states: "To be in relationship with the other (*autrui*) face to face is to be unable to kill" (p. 9).

Absolute alterity, for Levinas, concerns one's relation to the Other, who is "absolutely" other to the self. The Other cannot and must not be reduced to the same. Reducing the Other to the same, Levinas argues, is the root of "violence" (p. 13, 1996). Levinas claims: "Indeed, violence comes from opposition, that is to say, from the scission of being into Same and Other" (p. 13).

Like Kant's (2002) ethical imperatives, Levinas states that the self must not expect anything in return for *recognizing* the Other. The Other is my responsibility: what the Other does in return is none of my concern. Levinas (1985) states that the relation with the Other is "non-symmetrical" (p. 98). Levinas (1985) declares: "I am responsible for the Other without waiting for reciprocity" (p. 98). This is akin to the Buddhist idea that one must never expect anything from anyone or anything.

Levinas's Concept of Alterity

A crucial idea throughout Levinas's oeuvre is radical alterity (or radical difference). Levinas was a Holocaust survivor and understood all too well that authoritarian regimes reduce the Other to the same. In any kind of utopian society, difference gets wiped out. A society that engages in ethnic cleansing is one that reduces—through torture, murder or imprisonment—the Other to the same. The Holocaust was an attempt to reduce the Other to the same through mass murder and genocide. The Nazi plan was to erase difference through murder. Six million European Jews perished under the reign of the Third Reich. Six million more perished as well.

Alterity is a function of living systems, whether human or non-human animal. It is the diversity of species that protects life as a whole. Without a variety of species, without diversity of species, life as we know it would disappear. Decimated alterity means a decimated planet.

There is a legend—in Buddhist literature—about the search for the snow leopard: at bottom, this legend is about absolute alterity. The snow leopard is a rare animal who hardly ever shows his *face*. If one goes on a quest searching for the snow leopard, one will not find him. The story of the snow leopard signifies the liminal experience of alterity; this is an experience of looking but not finding. When one does not find that which one seeks, the phenomenology of lived alterity is at hand. The snow leopard represents that Other who can never be found and thus, never be reduced to the same. The quest to find the snow leopard—in actuality—is not about the snow leopard, literally; rather, it is a quest to find the self. To identify with the one who cannot be found is—psychologically—the quest to identify the Other with the self. This identification is a false one. The Other cannot be reduced to the self. Searching for the Other only to reduce the Other to the same means obliterating the Other.

Expect nothing, the Buddhist says to the seeker. Until the seeker understands this non-identification with the Other, his life will be little more than misery and suffering. Peter Matthiessen (1978) tells of his spiritual journey to find a snow leopard through his trek in Nepal. But before he leaves, his Buddhist teacher warns: expect nothing.

Matthiessen (1978)—who looks but does not find the snow leopard—learns "the not-looking-forward" to and "the without-hope-ness" (p. 300) of this quest. If you look, you shall not find. And what you look for is more about the *hope* of finding than the finding in and of itself.

I mention this Buddhist tale because it is akin to Levinas's (1985) lesson of "non-symmetrical" (p. 98) relationships. Levinas, too, argues that one should not expect anything from the Other. Only you are responsible for the Other. Do not look to identify with the Other because you will not find yourself in him. Expect nothing. As Kant (2002) reminds, doing a good deed is good in and of itself. If one expects a reward in return for doing something good, then one is not acting out of a sense of duty to the Other, but one is actually acting out of a selfish need to be rewarded for doing good deeds. That expectation and wish for a reward only points to self-interest.

In the context of Levinas, to expect something from the Other is to entertain delusion. The Other is not responsible for you or your happiness. The in-and-of-itself of the act and the duty to act only with the Other's best interest in mind should be enough, Kant stresses. The duty to the Other, the response to the Other and the responsibility for the Other should be enough. Thus both Levinas and Kant agree on these points.

Again, Levinas (1985) states that the relation to the Other—which is based on the *Face*—is not rooted in the "visual" (p. 88). Recall, the Face is a metaphor for God. For Levinas, "authentic relationship" (p. 88) is found in "discourse" (p. 88). Although Levinas was deeply rooted in the humanist tradition, a tradition that tended to ignore the non-human animal, one could make the connection to the non-human animal.In the context of this discussion, Levinas' ideas that relation to the Other are relevant. The snow leopard engages in a kind of discourse of not-being-present. The snow leopard signifies the not-said, the not-seen, the not-found. The snow leopard engages in a discourse of mystery; he is the sacred animal who hides his Face. The face of the Other is also found in the more-than-human, as David Abram (1996) might put it, or the Other-than—human. The face of the Other is, in fact, a cosmic face, something which Theologian Karl Rahner (1992) intimated in his work on theological anthropology.

Derrida, Alterity and Doing the Archiving

Alterity and archiving are interconnected. Archiving is an act of alterity. Archiving the past is always already about historicizing the Other. Alterity is the heart of archiving. Telling the story of the Other is not about the story of the same: the Other in the archive of the past is radically Other to the same. Archiving is inherently an ethical act to capture the past. The past is radical alterity in and of itself.

Archiving is an act of "response and responsibility" for both Levinas and Derrida. Drawing on Levinas, archiving is a sacred obligation. Derrida (1996) remarks that "The archive has always been a *pledge*, and like every pledge [gage], a token of the future.... what is no longer archived in the same way is no longer lived in the same way. Archivable meaning is also and in advance codetermined by the structure that archives" (p. 18). The *pledge* of archivization is a sacrosanct pledge.

The archive—although about the past—points towards the future. To study the past, to think philosophically about the archive of the past, is also to live it and project it into the future. What must be avoided is a mimetic archivization of the past, an archivization that is simply paraphrasing. To engage in philosophy—archivally—is to work with-and-in alterity, to work with-and-in altered spaces of time, place, geography and culture.

The archived past changes depending upon the way in which the archive is presented and re-presented. Derrida (1991) emphasizes the "plurivocity" (p. 46) of historicity. The historiography of the archive is always already, then: it is pluri-vocal. That is, history co-exists within simultaneous and multiple historiographies. Multiple archivizations occur at once, or at competing times, in parallel or in contradistinction. There is no one historiographical time, no one archive; rather, multiple stories unfold, some contradictory, some competing, some conflicting, some co-existing, some dis-connected and dis-orienting. Whatever the archive is, it is—in and of itself—radical alterity. Derrida (1976) writes that the

> The enigmatic model of the *line* is thus the very thing that philosophy could not see when it had its eyes on the interior of its own history. The night began to lighten a little at the moment when linearity—which is not loss or absence but the

repression of pluri-dimensional symbolic thought—relaxes its oppression because it begins to sterilize the technical and scientific economy that it has long favored. In fact for a long time its possibility has been bound up with that of economy, of thesaurization, of capitalization, sedentarization, hierarchization, of the formation of ideology by the class that writes or rather commands the scribes. (p. 86)

Derrida calls for "shocks" (p. 87) that break through linear thinking that serve to *sediment* ideology in order to present a neat and tidy history which—-in actuality—forecloses on the future. Derrida (1976) calls for the destruction of linear "models" of thought that serve only to control and constrain when, in fact, lived experience and the way it gets philosophically archived is much more complex. There is a politics involved in the way in which historiography gets written, the way in which archives get handed down throughout generations; we must read what comes before us with a critical lens. Gramsci (2000) warns that without criticality one can get "imprison[ed]" in a "pre-established schema" (p. 50) blinding one to the way "utopianism [becomes reified as] philistinism" (p. 49). Gramsci (2000) comments that "utopia is authority, not spontaneity" (p. 51). An archivization that pretends to be a closed system of thought erases the movements and shifts of the very architectonics of history-in-process. Hence, the work of the archive means process and fluidity. Derrida (1996) notes that "the archive is never closed" (p. 68); in fact, "[t]he archivist produces more archive" (p. 68). In other words, archives take on a life of their own. After the archive is thought through philosophically and historically, written down and published, another archivist takes up where the previous archive left off.

Archiving Catastrophes

Derrida's (1996) key text on the archive is subtitled *A Freudian Impression*. The catastrophe of the Freudian archivization—says Derrida—is the very erasure of Freud. The impression that Freud is irrelevant demonstrates only that he is, in fact, relevant. Freud's very erasure from the archive makes his re-appearance even uncanny. Freud taught that what we think we know we probably do not. What we think we remember, we probably do not. The catastrophe for Freud is the impression that he is no longer relevant. Freud is the specter that haunts academic psychology and the archivization of psychology in general. Freud is the return of the repressed. The more psychologists claim his irrelevance, the more he comes back to haunt. Freud is the *revenant* of psyche. Freud has left an indelible *impression* upon Western culture—no matter how much psychologists try to erase his influence.

Derrida (1978) troubles the notion of the archive and its related term archeology, drawing on the work of Foucault. Derrida (1978) comments:

> A history [referring to Foucault's *Archaeology of Knowledge*] that is, an archaeology against reason doubtless cannot be written, the concept of history has always been a rational one. It is the meaning of "history" or *archia* that should have been questioned first perhaps. A writing that exceeds, by questioning them, the values, the "origin," "reason," and "history" could not be contained within the metaphysical closures of archeology. (p. 36)

Perhaps an archive—the impression of remembrance, the call to remembrance, interrupts the faculty of reason. Archivization—as a call toward remembrance is not built on reason—rather it is built on sense *impression*. The senses and reason are, of course, related, but the senses are not the same as reason. An *impression* (Derrida, 1996) is built upon the dream and its repression. If anything, reason gets in the way of archiving remembrance because it serves as a form of censorship to remembrance. Remembrance, the *impression* that pains, that overwhelms, begs to be put under erasure. But the stronger the impression of erasure, the stronger—in turn- the force of unleashed repression. The return of the repressed upends reason.

Foucault was not Freudian. However, Foucault's (1972) *Archaeology of Knowledge* is—in reality—an *anarchy of knowledge*, for it is not logical or linear, but arbitrary. Derrida, in contradistinction to Foucault, is more sympathetic to the Freudian project. And ironically, the Freudian project is, in some ways, related to the anarchy of knowledge about which Foucault writes. The Freudian impression of the dream, remembrance and the archive—in and of itself—is subject to erasure and repression; it stands outside of reason and rationality. The Freudian impression, rather, is an anarchy of the senses.

Derrida's (1995) concern turns to the "abandoned archive" (p. 295). Likewise, Foucault's archaeology of knowledge is, in some ways, about what gets occluded, erased, upended, or falls outside of archeology to begin with. Knowledge-building is, Foucault argues, completely and utterly arbitrary. If *archive fever*— means anything at all—it means that the archive is impressed feverishly. The "abandoned archive" (Derrida, 1995, p. 295) is of great concern against the fever of the pandemic (covid-19). The pandemic is the impression of the fever forever etched in memory and must never be abandoned to the dustbin of history. Is it not our responsibility to archive the impression of the fever of covid-19? If not now, when? Hillel the Elder—ancient Talmudic scholar—asked. If not us, who? Who will be left after all is said and done? The future is unknowable. Now is the time to act, to write the archive, this feverish history.

Alterity and the Paradoxical Nature of Archivization

Derrida (1996)—drawing on psychoanalysis—points out that the process of archivization is paradoxical. The paradox of the archive makes archiving all the more difficult. Derrida states that Lacanian psychoanalysis

> Can tell us about these paradoxes of archivization, about its blanks, the efficacy of its details or its nonappearance, its capitalizing reserve or... about the radical destruction of the archive, in ashes, without the repression through a mere total displacement. (p. 44)

Whether the archive "appears" or not, emerges or not, makes an impression or not, is contingent, and dependent upon who tells the story to whom. Who has the right to destroy the archive? The "destroyed" archives are those stories forever lost in time and space.

The archive is more than dates, facts, things, and occurrences. Who writes the archives? Who *unwrites* the archives? Why stories of the archive emerge and/or disappear or why they never appear at all are political and psychological questions. What truths do we hide from the public at large? What is too much to take in emotionally and how can we capture catastrophic archivization without reducing it to either politics or psychology? Derrida points out that a remainder, a leftover, an image or impression is always already anticipating a future to come. Whatever is captured or left out, whatever memory-traces are left over—as Freud might put it—whatever can be gleaned from the "capitalizing reserve" (Derrida, 1996, p. 44) is always already something Other, it is always already Alterity at-hand or Alterity to-hand.

Catastrophic archivization is—paradoxically—beyond language, or understanding, beyond comprehension or reason, beyond signification. Catastrophic archivization ruptures and rips time, as Gilles Deleuze and Felix Guattari (2003) might put it. Deleuze and Guattari (2003) might also suggest that archivization is, in fact, *not narrative* at all. Catastrophic archivization shatters narrative altogether.

The to-come, as Derrida puts it, is Messianic time when catastrophic archivization begins. Benjamin (2016) writes of a "historical constellation" (p. 65) whereby images stand, or "standstill" (Benjamin, 2006, p. 43) outside of the everyday and perhaps are even—as Edmund Husserl might say—bracketed out of lived-time. "Messianic time" is not narrative. Archivization emerging in Messianic time, is about time. But Messianic time is not Bergson's smooth time of *duree*. Messianic time—the archivization of what is to come—is ripped time akin to the ripped fabric of the universe. Ripped time is subject to destruction, disappearance, mutation, and falling away. The catastrophic stories that are told through the process of archivization are subject to black holes, as it were, in memory, or are subject to falling into worm holes that move time backwards. Time is not one dimensional and does not flow smoothly. Nor does archivization. So, it is not just a question of arbitrary knowledge, as Foucault intimates. No, it is about much more than that.

Perhaps Messianic time and Levinas' metaphor of the Face of God—which is not based on visualization— collide in the duty and responsibility to archive. Again, archivization is not smooth narrative; it is gaps and holes, fissures and forgetfulness; and yet—the responsibility and response—as Levinas and Derrida might say—are of theological and philosophical necessity. Here, the theological and philosophical point towards an ethical obligation in a profanely-sacred sense—as in Eliade's (1957) *The Sacred and the Profane*—to archive that which is, ironically, unarchivable, paradoxical and utterly Other to lived experience as we know it.

Derrida (1978) claims—as against Levinas—that history [or its archivization] is not "totality" but "transcencendence" (p. 117). Derrida states:

> *Within history* which the philosopher cannot escape, because it is not history in the sense given to it by Levinas (totality), but it is the history of the departures from totality without which no totality would appear as such. History is not the totality transcended by eschatology, metaphysics, or speech. It is transcendence itself. (p. 117)

Counter to these claims, I argue that history—as archivization—is neither totality nor transcendence. Archivization is sacred—immanence located in the profane. Nor is Messianic time—as I understand it—transcendent. Messianic time is also sacred—immanence: it emerges in the "now time" as Walter Benjamin puts it. The "now time" is immanent even though things are still to come. However, the to-come is not a movement upward or away from the groundedness of being-in-time. Archivization—as historiography—is a plurality of movements that run hither and yon, haphazardly—but these movements do not transcend the groundedness in the here-and-now even if they imply a backward and forward motion in time. But the future is not a transcendence, which is the metanarrative of Christocentrism. Christendom—as Kierkegaard emphasized—is the lazy person's take on Christianity. Christendom is the Sunday churchgoer who has little idea that suffering and sacrifice make for Christian discipleship (as Dietrich Bonhoeffer would later put it). And in the face of catastrophes and horrors, pandemics and private tragedies, ignorance—in any form—including the ignorance of Christendom—will not do. Christendom does not understand the Messianic, for Messianic time is difficult; it is not the easy path taken by the lazy.

Messianic time for both Derrida and Benjamin—as something difficult to think—happens when things split open and break apart through immersion in the here and now. Messianic time is not rational. Rather it occurs—or happens—through images, impressions, intuitions and Otherness. Messianic time is Otherness; it is alterity. Messianic time is beyond explanation, exegesis or rationalization. Archivization is the very act of doing the work of the Messianic, of the to-come (as Derrida would put it).

Derrida (1978) remarks that "There is no experience which can be lived other than in the present" (p. 132). Yet the present is enwrapped in the past and the future. Derrida (1978) states:

> In Levinas.... In the living present... all temporal alterity can be constituted and appear as such: as other past present, other future present, other absolute origins relived in intentional modification... Only the actual unity of my living present permits other presents (absolute origins) from appearing as such, in what is called memory or anticipation. (p. 132)

Memory and anticipation of the future occur simultaneously or in a haphazard fashion. Anticipation is Messianic time, while memory is mostly repressed, forgotten or buried in multiple archives. Collective memories and anticipations complicate the matter further.

The most difficult anticipation is that of death. Derrida (1978) remarks that "The living present [shot through with both memory and anticipation] is originally marked by death" (p. 132). To anticipate paradise is to deny death; to anticipate paradise is to cover over the finality of death, the finitude of experience. Anticipation as Messianic time is the to-come, but the to-come is not, nor should it be, given over to false hope or piety; it should not be given over to a naïve concept like paradise, or heaven.

What is anticipated is the work, *the ethical work*, to be done in the name of archivization, the obligation to work in the archive even in the face of death, toward the face of the Other, not as a visual manifestation of the gaze, but as an ethical relationship without reciprocity—as Levinas maintains, a Kantian duty without expectation. Anticipation is duty without expectation; anticipation is an obligation without expecting anything in return. Anticipation is also the duty without expectation and obligation without reciprocity.

Death is finality. Death is finitude. Death is without anticipation because it just is. Death is death and no more than that. There is no afterlife after death. Even if there is an after-life, after death, one needs to live in the present in order to work for the past and the future in this life, in the here and now. The archivization of death is our ethical obligation while we are still standing, while we are still alive. Death is the ultimate alterity. One we cannot ever know or understand.

Archivization of death is alterity. Archivization of death does not reduce the Other to the same, nor does it reduce the past to the present, nor does it reduce the present to the future. The past-present-future are always already forms of alterity, forms of paradox, and in the end impossible to think. Just as death is impossible to think, the past-present-future are always already multiple, chaotic, aporetic and radically Other. They are mixed up together and half-forgotten, repressed and re-remembered differently at different times throughout collective recollection as well as individual recollection.

The Trace

Derrida's notion of the trace is a metaphor. It is a slippery metaphor; it is difficult to conceptualize perhaps because it is not exactly a concept, but an impression, an image, a sensation. The trace is not literally something that can be tracked or closed in upon itself. A trace is open to endless futurity, Derrida might say. A trace is akin to what Derrida calls a cinder. The cinders from a fireplace cannot be conceptualized; they fall from ashes, from fire, from glowing light, from dying light. The trace is what is left over after the free fall from logs burning or from the flames of the fire; the trace is a non-concept; no one can calculate or regulate, categorize or systematize the trace.

In the context of archivization, the trace is its own impossibility. The trace is topological, not chronological. The topological in Walter Benjamin's (1999)

Arcades Project—refers to the topology of cities: that cities are felt in lived-time as surfaces. Traces, topology, and the topological are but traces without centers, without places without perimeters.

The trace slips through grand metanarratives—such as Marx's *Manifesto*—as Derrida (1994) writes in *Specters of Marx*. Marx is a trace, a specter; his work is ghosted. In fact, Derrida points out that both Marx (1994) and Freud (1996) are traces, *revenants*, indelible hauntings. The polarizing figures of Marx and Freud mark the return of the repressed.

Neither is the trace predictable nor pre-ordained. Things do not have to happen the way that they do; nothing is inevitable in history. Historiography is the trace of unpredictable motion. Archivization is the historiography of the trace. Just when one attempts to say what the past was, it slips; the past leaves traces. Re-presentations are shifting markers of the past instantiated in the present. The future shifts depending upon how the past gets represented as traces of an unbearable to-come.

An unusable past is put to rest, erased, altered, or re-visioned so as to re-write a past that never was, in order to cover over what, in fact, was. As against Derrida's critics—who argues that his is a philosophy of radical relativism—Derrida is not arguing for any kind of post-truth. Derrida's philosophy is not a radical relativism, an anything goes philosophy. He never argues for the unusable past to be erased or altered. Derrida argues for the right to know the truth of what was, for justice, democracy, obligation and responsibility.

The archive and the trace are concepts that point to a more nuanced metaphysics. Derrida argues that the archive and the trace in the context of historicity—without origin, without reification—opens horizons to think historicity otherwise. Derrida (2002) states:

> Philosophy has never been the unfolding responsible for a unique, originary assignation linked to a unique language or to the place of a sole people. Under its Greek name and in its European memory, it has always been bastard, hybrid, grafted, mulilinear, and polyglot. We must adjust our practice of the history of philosophy our practice of history and of philosophy, to this reality. (p. 10)

Derrida's notions of archivization and the trace are—at root—steeped in notions of responsibility, politics and democracy. If anything, Derrida is a political philosopher, something about which Peter Trifonas (2002) has emphasized repeatedly. In fact, Trifonas states that for Derrida, "The question of the right to philosophy is precisely a question of democracy and the validity of its systems of governance"

(p. 90). Derrida (2002)—in *Echographies of Television*—stresses that one cannot do deconstruction without political "urgency"—and yes, in the midst of things that are ambiguous, what Derrida calls the undecideable—one must decide. And in fact, if no deliberation is at hand, ethicality cannot be had. This is not a new idea; in fact, deliberation and its ethicality can be traced back to the writings of Aristotle.

Derrida (1986) discusses the trace in the context of the history of metaphysics. The following citation, though difficult to unpack, suggests that the history of metaphysics—or one might say the archivization of that history—is not sedimented historiography. Who decides what metaphysics is? Who is left out of the traditional canon of the history of philosophy, of metaphysics, and why? The trace is a metaphor for the slips and folds—as Deleuze would put it—of archivization. There is no definitive history of philosophy and there is no definitive philosophy of history. Derrida (1986)—in *Margins of Philosophy*—says of metaphysics that

> it is not surrounded but rather traversed by its limit, marked in its interior by the multiple furrow of the margin. Proposing *all at once* [italics in original] the monument and the mirage of the trace, the trace simultaneously traced and erased, simultaneously living and dead, and, as always, living in its simulation of life's preserved inscription. (p. 24)

That which is left over, that which remains as a trace of history, what leaves traces, can be altered or even destroyed. But deconstruction, as Derrida repeatedly points out, is not destruction. Philosophy-as deconstruction—in my estimation—should not announce the death of metaphysics, although some call for this very death to occur. This annunciation of the death of metaphysics—is, in fact, violence done to an entire movement of thought. Although the history of metaphysics is in need of critique, it is not a question of its sheer destruction.

Michel Serres (1995) is highly critical of the violence to scholars done by the academy in general; both Serres and Derrida have always been critics of education systems that do violence to the scholar, especially scholars who commit to the Other of knowledges, and the knowledges of the Other. Both Derrida and Serres have been critics of the violence of the lack of ethicality—in honoring the work of the Other—in the arts, humanities and the sciences. Serres was a scientist who critiqued science from within his own profession. Serres, however, was not advocating anti-science, or post-truth. Serres (1983; 1995, e.g.)—like Derrida-—was a philosopher in search of the truth and the ethics of the truth, the truth of the multiple. In every discipline, critique is necessary. Science is in need of critique.

Philosophy is in need of critique. Education is in need of critique. Critique does not mean dismissal, though. Derrida and Serres are both fierce critics of universities in general. But again this does not mean that they did not benefit from being educated in universities; they both advocated for a new kind of university altogether. The university-to-come, Derrida argued, would be one without administrators. Derrida argued that despite the problems of the university—generally speaking—scholars can do their work in the very place that inhibits their work; in fact, that very inhibition of the work at hand opens passageways to new kinds of work, new kinds of critique. The present situation, though, is still, for the most part, the university *with* administrators, with too many administrators. The problem is not the administrator in his person—the problem is the entire idea of an administered culture, as Adorno (2008) pointed out. The more a culture is administered, the more the bureaucracy of administration gets in the way of the work at hand. The present—of this highly administered academic culture—though, does not always have to be what it is: a future where there is room to think—minus a highly administered academia—could become a real possibility, some day. Or perhaps not. But who knows what the future holds? Nothing is pre-ordained; things can be otherwise. Let us hope that highly administered academic cultures are but a trace of things past.

Derrida (1986) states, "Since the trace is not a presence but the simulacrum of a presence that dislocates itself, displaces itself, refers itself, it properly has no site—erasure belongs to its structure" (p. 24). The notion of presence, which is highly problematic for Derrida, is in inverse relation to the trace. Derrida (1976) states:

> To confine writing to a secondary and instrumental function: translator of a full speech that was fully *present* (present to itself, to its signified, to the other, the very condition of the theme of presence in general), technics in the service of language, *spokesman,* interpreter of originary speech itself shielded from interpretation. (p. 8)

The assumption is that if Socrates were present, his presence makes him real. The unreality of a dead man, a dead Socrates, and the traces of his utterances makes his utterances less real. But does that make Socrates' dialogs any less important because he is no longer alive? No. Socrates—as a dead man—can no longer utter things in the presence of others. It is the case, though, that his utterances can be misheard and readers might—in fact—get him wrong. But interpretation is always open to misinterpretation. However, even if Socrates were still alive, listening to him pontificate in the streets of Athens does not necessarily mean that what is heard is actually what Socrates meant. Because someone is present—pontificating—does not necessarily mean that we understand him. In fact, the word that gets written down—and becomes part of the archive—might be better understood later, as time passes; for thought and understanding take time. But the history of philosophy, Derrida tells us, has actually been about about the end of writing, or ending the task of writing. When the correct answer is gotten no more philosophizing is necessary; no more writing is necessary. This is what Wittgenstein (1922) believed, at least in his early work, in his *Tractatus*. He felt that his was the final word—or so he thought at the time—on truth in philosophy. But after some time, Wittgenstein recanted this position. Later in 1958 in *Philosophical Investigations*—where he started all over again—again he believed that he answered all possible philosophical questions, thus ending the need for any more philosophical writing. But neither the *Tractatus* nor the *Philosophical Investigations* ended philosophy argumentation and conversation; in fact, both of these texts only raised more questions, and, in turn, more questions led to more writings—commentaries—that again only raised more questions, and in turn, more writings. Commentators, in fact, are still writing about Wittgenstein's work. And this will go on interminably, not only about Wittgenstein, but about anything that is written—that is worth its salt—that demands thought and rethought. Whether the writer is actually present or absent, dead or alive, more questions are raised, more writing emerges. All is open to interpretation, to writing; interpretations can never get at what the writer intended exactly. The more the questions a work poses, the more the questions get raised. The more the questions get raised, the more the problems get posed. Writing continues endlessly.

Derrida's other important point—in relation to this discussion—is that writing is not, in fact, "secondary" to speech: it is, indeed, intertwined with it. That the speaker might be present does not guarantee that what he says will be understood by others. Even if the writer is alive and tells you exactly what (he or she) means, even (he or she) does not always know exactly what (he or she) is saying. Philosophers are not fully conscious of what it is they are writing or saying.

The Freudian Impression is at hand: speech and writing are inter-twined, confused, confusing, unclear, meaning is never exact; what is said or written is perhaps not even what the speaker or writer intends. The unconscious drives much of the writing, *the mystical writing pad,* as Freud called it. The mystical suggests that one is never wholly in charge of what one is saying, doing or writing. There is a kind of mystical Otherness to all of these processes because they are driven by the unconscious. The writing—and the speech that is always already embedded in the writing—takes on its own life outside of the writer's conscious awareness. The reader, too, engages in transference and/ or mimesis when attempting to interpret texts. Sometimes the reader reads for what he already knows while ignoring what he cannot understand, or perhaps he misunderstands everything he reads. The reader, in a way, re-writes or even un-writes what he reads and re-interprets the text so as to write a new text through his interpretation or misinterpretation.

The greatest problem in academe is that scholars are taught to mimic what others say, imitate the jargon, repeating what it is that a writer has already said. The paraphrase is the absurdity—and problematic of academic work. Paraphrasing is not what intellectual labor should be. But the explication of the text sometimes gets in the way of the analysis and in fact too much paraphrasing (especially in the social sciences) overshadows analysis to the detriment of movement within a field of study. As Christopher Fynsk (1991) argues, there comes a time when a scholar must "abandon the commentator's position of relative safety" (p. viii). Thinking is not paraphrasing; thinking means moving away, veering off in analysis to explore one's own take on things. Thinking takes courage. Thinking means taking risks. Heidegger once asked whether we are able to think at all. And he once profoundly asked the question: what is this (thing) called thinking? Heidegger intimates that people cannot, in fact, think. And thinking is not something that can be taught either. This was Socrates' point. There is a vast difference between someone installed in a university and a true thinker. Being installed in a university—as a professor—does not necessarily make for a thinker.

In dictatorial countries, like Russia, students are taught to mimic, to memorize and repeat what it is that philosophers say. To question the very foundation of the university and or the government is to end up in prison, or gulags. Artists, educators, activists and film-makers—for example—who have attempted to think, to question, and to work outside of the accepted Russian narrative have ended up exiled or dead. Andrey Tarkovsky, film-maker, who was eventually exiled from Russia, dared to paint a portrait of a gloomy Russia, haunted by war, nuclear accidents and oppression. Is the United States soon to follow in dictatorial fashion? Who knows what the future holds? But I, for one, am not hopeful that democracy will hold in the present moment and the near future-to-come. The United States is slipping closer and closer to dictatorship. And this means the death of freedom and thought. And worse.

From cinema, Deleuze (1986; 1989) states, philosophical concepts emerge. It is here that questioning begins. To question state oligarchs, through the arts, education or philosophy, means risking life. Those who sell out to the State are rewarded, but pay out in other ways. Selling out means selling one's soul. Some argue that this is, in fact, what composer Dmitri Shostakovich did. But this is debatable. This composer wrote for the state, seemingly glorifying war and state-sponsored terrorism. It is not lost on one Julian Barnes (2016) that Shostakovich sold out. Barnes (2016), in *The Noise of Time,* begins the story of Shostakovich, with a suitcase in hand, waiting. He knew they would eventually come for him, the Soviets would eventually find him. Just one mistake, one slip, one comment, one critique could land one in a gulag. In time, Shostakovich's reputation suffered world-wide. Today, his reputation has been soiled. He is indelibly marked by collusion with the Soviet State. Shostakovich, like the German composer Carl Orff—dubbed Hitler's musician—colluded with the Third Reich, all in the name of fame and glory. Both Shostakovich and Orff have tainted legacies. Artists who sell out to state terror—for fame and glory—play their part in propping up dictators. Artists who misuse the muse(s)—if you will—for their own political gain are no better than Mephistopheles. This was Goethe's point; this was Thomas Mann's point. To dance with the devil is to play with fire.

Differance

Archivization, the trace and differance are all inter-related concepts for Derrida. Differance is perhaps the most Freudian of Derrida's concepts. Derrida (1976) states *"differance,* an economic concept [which designates]… the production of differing/deferring" (p. 23). Differance means both to differ and delay meaning. That which is deferred comes later. A deferred payment means to pay later. A deferred meaning suggests belated understanding. Or, sometimes Derrida suggests that meaning or understanding might not come at all.

The concept of differance also suggests radical alterity—radical difference—in the spirit of Levinas. This is why—I argued at the outset of this chapter that—Derrida is indebted to the work of Levinas; one can see traces of Levinas throughout Derrida's work, especially with the concepts of alterity, response and responsibility. Derrida, especially in the conceptualization of his notion of differance, frames alterity in a more Freudian way than Levinas.

Freud suggested that because of psychic defense mechanisms—e.g., denial and repression—meanings are always already delayed. Or, if repression is strong enough, meanings disappear from consciousness altogether. Repetition compulsion, acting out, reversals, reaction-formation and even hysteria—an unfortunate word—or what Freud (1953) also called conversion disorder—whereby psyche-somatic illnesses have no physiological cause—erupt belatedly on the scene. For Derrida radical alterity is more akin to Freud's ideas than Levinas' notion of alterity.

Further, I want to argue that differance could also become belatedly attached to allegory—meaning that stories stand for things outside of themselves, outside of narrow, literal parameters; differance-as-allegory points to broader meanings not initially intended. Differance-as-allegory, then, doubles Derrida's delayed and deferred deconstruction, taking on doubled-meaning, that this means that, that means something else and so forth.

But still, there is always the chance that meaning is not made at all, or not yet, or perhaps never. Thus, Derrida's notion of differance is more complicated than Levinas' notion of alterity, although alterity is certainly folded into the meaning of differance as well. Derrida's notion of differance takes meaning into multitudinous directions at once simultaneously; or, conversely the end result of differance could mean that no meaning is made at all, or the meaning that is made is never understood. Differance always includes its opposite, it can be dialectic or not, but it is always, as Derrida puts it, aporetic. Differance is always a question-to-hand. Derrida takes Levinas' concept of radical alterity to its extreme.

Plato's *Pharmakon*, about which Derrida writes, is not about the pharmacy per se. The *Pharmakon* is allegorical. Of course the *Pharmakon*, for Plato, concerns the ways in which medicines can serve as both poison(s) and/ or cure(s). Differance points to a both—and, not an either/or, as Kierkegaard (1987) would have it. This-and-that (as opposed to this or that) is a way of suggesting that things are not *monolingual*—to use Derrida's term—things are not monolithic; the this-and-that always already goes beyond singular meaning. Derrida's work, as a whole, questions the political ramifications of the resultant dualisms that occur out of universals (i.e., speech and writing, mind and body) that have created numerous problems for philosophy.

Today it is very difficult to defend universals or universalisms which nearly always end up as dualistic concepts—the very thing that philosophy has reified over centuries. Although Etienne Balibar (2020), in his work on *Universals*, attempts to defend universals with qualifications, I find his arguments unconvincing. Qualifying universals still does not justify what it is they set out to do: push further to the margin the multifarious voices on the edges. Perhaps mine is a misreading, but it seems to me that Balibar attempts to do the impossible. Universals can no longer maintain their hegemonic status. Derrida's project is—as I see it—completely counter to the defense of universals. Like Michel Serres, Deleuze and Guattari, multiples (that belie dualisms and universals) make more sense; Otherness and differance, alterity and voices from the margins put dualisms and universals into question. The ancient arguments of the One and the Many have come back to haunt traditional philosophers (see for instance, pre-Socratics such as Thales who argued that the universe is made up of the *One* element which is the essence of the universe versus Heraclitus who argued that the universe is made up of the many things that are continually in flux. (in Kaufman, 1968)).

The argument for universals begs the question, universal for whom? What do the universal concepts of freedom, liberty, fraternity, community mean? Who decides who has a right to freedom, liberty, fraternity and community? Notions of the East and the West must be re-thought as they always already beg the question of Orientalism, as Edward Said (1978) so eloquently pointed out. Deconstruction—which is not a method but, rather, a way to see the world anew, a new way to live as a philosopher even— overturns that which is unthought and perhaps taken-for-granted. Deconstruction—as a way to live a philosophical life—attempts to live-on within radical alterity. Universals perhaps unwittingly—perpetuate the erasure of marginalized voices—that do not fit within universal parameters of what counts as Western philosophy—for example. Writings from what used to be called the other Europe (or so-called marginal literatures from Eastern Europe, such as those of Kafka) or writings from the Other Americas, the Americas beyond the United States tend to get erased (so-called marginalized literatures, such as those of Gloria Anzaldua, who coined the phrase mestiza consciousness).

Deconstruction as a way of living-on (to use Derrida's phrase) in the world as a philosopher means living outside the limits of philosophy; deconstruction means pointing beyond traditional philosophical discourse; opening new avenues for doing philosophy, differently.

In another sense, differance, means "deferring" (1976, p. 23) or waiting. Derrida, like Benjamin, adds a Messianic dimension to his work. In other words, differance means to defer, to wait, to delay. After the biblical prophet Elijah, who has not yet come, neither has democracy, Derrida says. In *Echographies* (2002), Derrida states:

> And the *arrivant* [italics in the original] may always not come, like Elijah. It is the always-open hollow of this possibility, that is, in non-coming [*non-venue*, italics in the original], absolute disappointment [*deconvenue*] that I have a relation to the event: it is what may always not take place, too. (p. 14)

There is a waiting, an anticipation into an open future, never foreclosed by objectives, aims, destinations. And in this waiting, that which for which one waits, might never come and yet one still waits. The deferred event might not happen. This is Messianic time. And perhaps it is no accident that both Derrida and Benjamin draw upon the notion of the Messianic from the Hebrew Scriptures, as both philosophers were Jewish, although neither of them claimed to be religious. But in the Jewish tradition, Messianism—as it is especially linked to Elijah—haunts these thinkers; the Messianic is the specter for both Derrida and Benjamin. Elijah is the *revenant,* who haunts both Derrida and Benajmin.

The absence of closure is part and parcel of the work of both Derrida and Freud. A text—like life—does not result in closure; the text like life, is never fully understood. There is always a remainder, a left-over, a yet-to come. These left overs are, perhaps, unconscious. Especially in this connection, Derrida (1986) states that differance (that results in left-overs, in unconscious remainders) is "tied to Freudian theory" (p. 18). Recall, what is at stake for Derrida is the problem of presence, the problematization of the "presence as consciousness" (p. 18). Derrida's larger project is to interrupt the notion of presence. The presence of Socrates, again, does not make his words any more understandable. In fact, Socrates' very presence could, ironically, make his words even more confusing.

Further, Derrida's project is absolutely counter to Descartes; to the Cartesian scientific method, to Descartes' quest for certainty and indubitable principles. Derrida's project is counter to Cartesian rationalism, as well as Hume's empiricism. The problem with empiricism, Derrida points out, is that it is too becomes *vulgar.* In other words, empiricism too easily reduces what is complex to what is simple. Foucault—is in agreement with Derrida on this point—as he would later say that what you see is not what you think you see. Just because you look at something does not mean you understand what it is you are looking at. Both Foucault and Derrida caution that empirical research as it has been traditionally conceived, is highly problematic. Unlike Kant, Derrida does not wish to mend broken fences by attempting bridge rationalism and empiricism into a kind of transcendentalism. That too, for Derrida, is a failed project. Derrida seeks something radically different from rationalism, empiricism and Kant's transcendental bridge building.

Deconstruction is not unlike what many American Pragmatists had been calling for in the early 20th century: anti-foundationalism. The meaningless philosophical problems of epistemology—how we know what we know—must be re-thought against the backdrop of wars, violence and genocide.

The Pandemic and Derrida's Concepts

One can see how Derrida's concepts that I have briefly outlined in this chapter—namely, the archive, the trace and differance—lend themselves to grappling with the current pandemic we are living through. Covid-19 is raging on in ever new hosts. It is the parasite, about which Michel Serres (2007) writes, that has turned into a global killing machine. Archiving this horror is all the more important not only for the now but for the future-to-come. It is our responsibility to archive what we are living through now, so as to not let this pandemic slip from memory. Moreover, to archive the pandemic in lived-time, especially by those of us who have witnessed—first-hand—the ravages of the disease that is covid-19 has never been more important. We cannot afford not to archive this pandemic, this plague, this monster because the way we see the future depends upon the way in which this current horror gets documented. Future pandemics will occur, of course. But perhaps if we write and document and archive what is happening in the now, the future-to-come may in some way learn from what it is that we struggled through; perhaps in the very act of archivization of this pandemic, we can learn from the mistakes made along the way in not being able to stop the beast earlier.

But more than that this archivization is an ethical obligation to honor the dead. Testimony is our obligation—our response and responsibility—to those who lost their lives to the pandemic. To let the task of archivization slip by is to risk having revisionists unwrite this history, re-write it out of existence or explain it away.

The difficulty of archiving the pandemic is that it is ever in flux, it is ever changing and completely ravaging the globe. Who is next? How long do we have? What is life in the face of death? What is a life, after all, if it is not lived as a life worth living? When does the quality of life disappear? And then what? And what does it mean to witness the death of the Other? What does it mean to witness the trace of the Other's last breath? What does it mean to witness the trace of corpses piling up in refrigerator trucks?

Philosophers have been writing at a distance about death—-unless they have faced their own mortality—for as long as philosophy has been in existence. But to face death squarely in the face, to face one's own mortality, to witness the death of the Other, to struggle with the disease of covid, to know from the inside what this horror feels like? These are all serious philosophical questions and problems we must archive and trace in the now, before slipping into the nothingness of a future-of-no-future. There is an urgency to this writing, to this archivization, to the trace of life that is passing before us, to the trace of death that confronts all of us.

Philosophy and education might seem strange bedfellows but perhaps not. Curricular questions are, at root, philosophical ones. Teachers, and professors, students are all suffering from this pandemic; some are dying. School bus drivers are dying. School children are dying. Professors are dying. College students are dying. Is this not our concern? Should this not be, as Paul Tillich (1970) put it, our *ultimate* concern? Those who write at a distance about the unthinkable or the unbearable are now, perhaps *living* the unthinkable or the unbearable.

Curriculum studies, philosophy and education writ-large are all bedfellows, strange or not. It is time that we come together, work together to archive, to trace and to make certain that the future is not without our archivization. We may have our differences, indeed. And differance—as in the delayed and deferred meanings between and across disciplines—might thicken, not simplify—our phenomenological experiences, as we all must tell our stories, as unbearable as they might be.

We must not stand on the outside of this tragedy. We must not be sheltered in our safe spaces—if we are lucky enough to have them. None of us, at the end of the day, is sheltered from this horror. And if we remain locked up in our heads, refusing to engage in these discussions and deliberations about the now and the future that we might not even have, we are not paying homage to our own callings. None of us should feel privileged or above the fray. If we do, we have surprises waiting for us down the road. As Adorno (2008) strongly stated, philosophy—and I would add education and curriculum studies—must point to its other, to the non-conceptual. Living through a pandemic is living through the non-conceptual. But, still concepts are necessary in order to theorize that which is non-conceptual. Adorno (2008) argued that no matter what our disciplines may be, our obligation as intellectuals concerns widening narrow parameters or academic fiefdoms in order to better to face head on what is right in front of us.

Those of us who have lived on the precipice of death know all too well that life is not forever; it is a gift, and we are but a blip in time. Christopher Fynsk (1991) cites Blanchot on death as he states: "exposure to death, no longer my own exposure, but someone else's, whose living and closest presence is already the eternal and unbearable absence, an absence that the travail of deepest mourning does not diminish.... It is with that absence—its uncanny presence, always under the prior threat of disappearing" (p. xvii) to which we must attend.

I have witnessed many people die needlessly from covid-19; I have watched many take their last and final breaths. I have witnessed the horrors of the families left behind, attempting to cope with the tragic life that has been lost. I have seen too much. And it is too much to bear. This writing is a testament to those who have perished. This archivization is not by any means a mere exercise in abstract concepts and philosophy at a distance. I have been on the front lines, I am a chaplain and I am a professor. But I am also part of history and have the responsibility to tell the unbearable stories that I have witnessed. I have also been a victim of covid, not once but twice. And I do not know how much longer I have on this planet. None of us knows this. This is why I write with urgency. Because the moment is now. The future is our responsibility, no matter how much we stumble and even get it wrong.

Some might argue that the philosophical concepts I have presented have little meaning in the face of the pandemic. Some might argue that working their way through abstractions is too much work, too hard, too difficult. Why is it that I simply do not get to the point? Some might ask. Why should I not simply tell literal stories? My argument in this book is that stories do not simply stand on their own. They demand conceptualization and interpretation. We have little understanding of a story without interpretation and theorization. But contrarily, it is not enough to theorize without making the abstract concrete. This tightrope we walk as scholars is difficult. And I intend to keep the difficulty in this text.

The archive, the trace and differance are all slippery concepts. We must take care to not reify any of these. The archive is not one thing. There is not one archive. Archivization is not one thing. Archivization is historicity, it is the history of archiving something. Historicity-as-archivization is movement and process. Archivization does not mean anything goes either. This is not an escape hatch for radical relativism. The very act of archivization—because it does imply doing, gathering, collecting, sorting through, editing, corresponding, upending, turning things on their head, moving backwards and looking to the future makes this a very difficult project.

Hospitals, universities, schools, corporations and social media have turned covid into a paint by numbers game. The numbers of dead do not tell the story. Rather, they erase the humanness of the story. They only make us numb to the story. Concealing the truth, cooking up the lies about covid must be called out. The search for the truth is the task at hand. I take Foucault's (2011) notion of the *courage of truth* to heart. But the truth is hard to grasp because the truth of the pandemic is ever-changing, always in motion. It is very difficult to capture a moving object.

The trace, Derrida's slippery concept, is useful especially in the context of archivization and truth-telling. To trace the truth of the matter, the truth of the pandemic as it is continually in flux, continually changing is no easy task. The truth is a moving object; the truth is the very stream of history; but this stream is not smooth, or linear, or clear. The trace of the truth of the pandemic is non-conceptual, completely illusive but demands conceptualization and theorization. The trace is akin to Derrida's notion of cinders; those burning embers that are left over after a fire, forever moving, drifting out of sight. The trace of the pandemic is everywhere and nowhere; the virus is invisible; it is a cinder, an ember, an invisible terror that kills. This virus—this killer—is not something one can see; it is a whiff of death floating from a trauma bay, a trace of the finality of things, the final goodbye is but a trace, the body tossed into the morgue only leaves a trace of the human zipped up in a body bag. The trace lingers in the corpse, the dead body.

Covid kills: in the end the trace of blue feet is all that is left, because moments after death occurs the feet do, in fact, turn blue. That blue color it is but a trace of the human, gone forever. It is easier to gloss over the real: our thoughts and prayers are with you, all will be well, things will get better. These are but ridiculous words that are not only meaningless but psychologically damaging. These are not the words of truth; these are the gloss of lies. Truth comes hard.

In the quest for the truth, the truth of the matter is that—at this juncture in history—we do not understand what it is that we are living through. Derrida's notion of differance points to the delay and deferral of meaning. Derrida says we might understand things later, or perhaps never. The child who is left by himself after his parents die; the parents who lose their child to covid cannot process what has happened. These unnecessary deaths are cruel and meaningless.

The slipperiness of language leaves us speechless in a world where all that once made sense no longer does. Our senses lie, our reason falters. Yet we must pursue the truth of this pandemic through a continual archivization. This book is only a beginning. The task at hand will never be finished. How to get a hold of the stream of historicity in the midst of horror.

The philosopher's stone, they say, is death. Philosophy is the preparation for death. Death is the cornerstone of philosophy. It is an idea one ponders. It is the key idea throughout the history of philosophy and yet none of us understands what death means. It is one thing to ponder death—philosophically. It is another thing altogether to witness the death of a child, a mother, a father, a sister, a brother. It is another thing altogether to live through the horrors of a pandemic. The unbearable thought of final goodbyes is just that: unbearable. This book is about that which is unbearable.

4

Thomas Merton's Crisis of The Unspeakable

Thomas Merton's theology pushes thought beyond what thought can think. Merton's theology embraces the *via Negativa*. Merton performs, theologically, what Adorno (2005) calls "negative truth" (p. 50). Negative truth is, indeed, that which is awful. Merton's theology is relevant to our current era. We are living in the awfulness of the era of the pandemic called covid-19. It is as if Merton (1966) is speaking to us now as he states: "One of the awful facts of our age is the evidence that it is stricken indeed, stricken to the very core of its being by the presence of the unspeakable" (p. 5). The era before us, upon us and seemingly never leaving us, is, indeed, the "age" of the "presence of the unspeakable" (Merton, 1966, p. 5). The pandemic is not local problem, it is a global one. It is a problem not of a state or a nation, but it is a problem that the world shares. Unfortunately, this is the state of the world community: if there is one thing we all have in common, it is the commons-of-covid. The utter horrors of covid—in all of its multitudinous variations, its multi-variants—is devastating populations everywhere. Gabriel Marcel (1950) writes:

> We must admit the extreme probability that we are heading for catastrophes even more terrible, even more uprooting, than those which many of us have witnessed during the last thirty-five years. (p. 166)

Marcel was concerned—in the 1950s—about more terrible catastrophes to come. Well, unfortunately he was right. Covid is that more horrible catastrophe that is here. Marcel's predictions were unfortunately prescient.

How can religion survive in the face of continual catastrophe? More often than not, the religion of lay persons is that of gloss, of covering over hard truths, of painting death as if it does not really happen, because the after-life is to come. Let me make it clear here that theology is not religion. Theology is the conceptualization of the spiritual; yes, sometimes it can become dogmatic. But there are workable theologies, like Marcel, like Merton, who were both realistic theologians, theologians who sought truth in a terrible world. Neither glossed over the horrors that they witnessed during their lifetimes, or used theology as a crutch.

Nietzsche eschewed moralizing; he detested Christianity as it got played out by Sunday Church goers. Religion can become a very dangerous game, indeed. It has been used historically to marginalize and harden hatreds. But in this chapter I work through theology, Merton's theology, which might help us to think through what Merton calls the "unspeakable."

Theology used to be considered the crowning discipline of the university. No longer. Now theology is considered a useless discipline; it is ghettoized in seminaries. As an academic discipline, theology is in trouble. The concept of God is in trouble. Who needs a God who allows the horrors of this pandemic to kill millions? Where is God when a mother's child needlessly dies from covid-19? Where is God when a child's parents are both lost to covid? And yet, people want to believe that there is a God. And yet, people want the chaplain to baptize their child before they go to the next world, wherever they think that might be. In fact, some parents are so frantic before the imminent death of a child that if the chaplain does not arrive on time to baptize the child before death, the parents believe that their child could go to hell. What kind of a cruel theology is that? God is dead. The child is dead. Theology is dead. Nietzsche was right. But perhaps Merton and theologians like him can help to resuscitate workable theologies? Theology, like philosophy, is the systematic study of concepts related to religious beliefs and rituals. There is more to theology than the concept of God. But, still what about this God? This god who is merciful? Is he?

Merton (2007)—the trappist monk who doubted himself at every step of the way—who doubted God, who doubted his calling, who doubted whether or not taking vows was even the right thing for him to do, did not doubt God's existence in the end and yet seemed tormented by the evil he witnessed in the world. Merton was a fierce critic of the Vietnam War, he saw the cruelties of war, the needless and violent deaths of war. He knew all too well at death the clock stops: "No clock, only the heart's blood, only the word" (p. 133).

Merton (1955) states: "There are times, then, when in order to keep ourselves in existence at all we simply have to sit back for a while and do nothing" (p. 123). Doing nothing, for Merton, did not mean, however, not being engaged politically. Perhaps Merton meant that stillness in the midst of chaos is necessary to get one's bearings. Unlike many monks—who feel that their work is in prayer only—Merton was an activist and a writer. Many monks are cloistered in abbeys; they believe that prayer is their work. Merton loved prayer as well but he was also adamant that the monastic life did not exclude the political. But in order to engage the political—contemplation and study are necessary in order to engage in political action that does not become reactionary. Acting without thinking is reactionary.

Merton also argued that getting distance from the world becomes necessary in order to engage in the world. Merton became a Trappist Monk. This is ironic because trappist monks take a vow of silence. But Merton felt compelled to write; indeed, he spoke through his writing. Writing is a form of political activism, some say. And yet, he was tormented by these competing callings. Merton's (1966) contradictory life puzzled him so. He felt that it was his calling to become a Trappist Monk taking the vow of silence; while, on the other hand Merton felt called to write, in order to speak the unspeakable, to be in the "presence of the unspeakable" (p. 5) to "raid" (p. 1) "the unspeakable" (p. 5).

Merton's (1966) book *Raids on the Unspeakable*, although written during the upheavals of the Vietnam War, still resonate with that which is unspeakable in the context of the covid pandemic. The "raids" of the "unspeakable"—those unspeakable and unbearable stories of living through this pandemic need to be written, to be archived. The "unspeakable" "raids" on untimely deaths must be spoken. As Derrida often pointed out speech and writing are not two things; they are intertwining activities. Derrida says that speech is always already in writing.

Thomas Merton (1966) writes about the necessity of pessimism. Merton's theology is a pessimistic theology. Matthew Fox (1995) points out that theology is not all light, that theology should not become theology lite. In fact, Fox warns that theology that is shrouded in too much light—ironically—presents certain dangers. Fox states that cults are shrouded in too much light. Marshall Applewhite the guru of Heaven's Gate—a cult shrouded in too much light—convinced his followers that they would be better off on what he called the away team; he convinced his disciples that the away team would fly them up to heaven.

This cult ended in tragedy as many cult members died by suicide. This was a cult of all light and ended badly.

Augustine certainly did not espouse an all light theology, nor did St. Paul, nor did St. John of the Cross. Martin Luther—the Protestant Reformer—did not engage in an all light theology either. The priesthood of believers who engage in stripped-down rituals, enter the starkness of Lutheran churches, as a reminder that being a true Christian is hard, not easy; the way of the cross is not light, it is heavy. Like Martin Luther, Soren Kierkegaard (1973; 1854-1855) stressed the trials and sacrifices of becoming a true Christian. His *Attacks upon Christendom—* is a condemnation against what he considered to be the mediocrity of Christianity; Kierkegaard railed against the Sunday Church goer who was not only hypocritical, but did not understand Christianity at all. The Sunday Church goer—Kierkegaard inimated—does not understand what Isaiah's suffering servant meant, what the Christian gospel really meant.

The *pieta*—the dying god in the mother's arms—is hardly light fare. Some theologians claim that the pieta is the centerpiece of true Christianity. The suffering Christ on the cross, bleeding and mocked is central to Christianity. Christ cries out, why hast thou forsaken me, abba? Father where art thou? But Kierkegaard tells us that Christendom has forgotten the central tenets of true Christianity. Christianity is a religion that embraces suffering and sacrifice; suffering, for Kierkegaard, is the heart of Christianity. Suffering is the *via negativa*. Kierkegaard (1988) argued that the true Christian must endure difficult *Stage[s] on Life's Way*. It is ironic that Kierkegaard—the deeply religious Christian—and Nietzsche (2010)—who called himself the Anti-Christ—are not dissimilar. Both hated mediocrity, both hated false piety. It is a "difficult across"— Nietzsche (1999) says of *Zarathustra*—life is a "tightrope" walk, life is akin to hanging over an abyss.

Matthew Fox became an Episcopalian Priest after being ex-communicated from the Catholic Church. Catholic priests cannot veer from Catholic dogma. Catholic priests are not protected by academic freedom—even if they are installed in universities. This is one reason—some argue—that Catholic theology has lagged behind Protestant theology, academically (This is a debatable point because there is much in Catholic theology which is quite impressive. e.g. the work of Karl Rahner, 1992). Censorship of Catholic Priests and the threat of ex-communication if one veers from the Pope's mandates does little to encourage generativity or creativity.

Although Thomas Merton was outspoken and a fierce critic of the Vietnam War, he managed not to get ex-communicated. During the Second Vatican

Council—especially during the 1960s—the Church took a liberal turn. But the Catholic Church—with the exception of the Second Vatican Council—has been and remains politically reactionary.

Merton's Courage of Truth

Throughout this book I have come back to Foucault's (2011) notion of the courage of truth; the willingness to die for the truth, in the spirit of Socrates. There are not many who are willing to die for the truth. But Thomas Merton was. And perhaps he did, although the cause of his death is still debated.

Merton's *courage of truth*—to draw on Foucault's (2011) words—was evident in his willingness to not gloss over things. Merton asks: "Is it pessimism to diagnose cancer as cancer? Or should one simply go on pretending that everything is getting better every day" (p. 72)? To go on pretending that things are getting better, or that the cancer will just disappear on its own is little more than magical thinking. To face, head on, a diagnosis of cancer is beyond the thinkable. But thinking the unthinkable, bearing the unbearable is necessary, if one is a truth-seeker.

Should a physician lie to a patient who suffers from terminal cancer? Or is it better to tell the truth? Adorno (2005) would say that "negative truth" (p. 50) must be faced, encountered and confronted. Giving terminal cancer patients false hope is little more than cruelty. Consoling patients who suffer from terminal cancer is nothing short of criminal. In fact, physicians—at least today—are bound by their oath to truth-telling; they must square with their patients. It should be noted, though, that in past decades this was not always the case. Physicians sometimes lied to their patients who suffered from terminal illness because it was thought that that was the kinder, gentler path.

False piety, false hope, "sentimental"... "mushy spiritual reading"... and "consolations" (1972, p. 247), Merton exclaims do not lead to what is deeply theological. For Merton, the deeply theological, the *via Negativa,* a theological tradition that can be traced back to St. John of the Cross (2017), attempts to grapple with the edges of lived experience, the devastations of catastrophes, the unanswered questions about needless suffering and deaths. St. John of the Cross—who lived in the 1500s—best exemplifies this theological tradition. Profound theology leads

> not to the easiest, but to the most difficult;
> not to the most delightful, but to the most distasteful;

not to the most gratifying, but to the less pleasant;
not to what means rest for you, but to hard work;
not to the consoling, but to the unconsoling. (2017, p. 149)

St. John of the Cross (2017) stressed the necessity of entering "the dark night through which the soul journeys" (p. 114). It is here that one confronts the unspeakable, the unthinkable, the catastrophic. And it is here that true Christianity can be found. If one is Christ's disciple, suffering is a theological imperative.

To minimize the suffering of a parent who loses a child in a mass shooting, to minimize the suffering of a child who loses a parent to covid-19 helps no one. Meaningless consolations are not good medicine for the psyche. In medicine, the physicians' creed is do no harm. However, when one resorts to niceties, cliches and sentimentality, much harm is done. Nietzsche (1997) states that

> The Greeks likewise differed from us in the evaluation of *hope:* they felt it to be blind and deceitful; Hesiod gave the strongest expression to this attitude in a fable whose sense is so strange no more recent commentator has understood it—for it runs counter to the modern spirit, which has learned from Christianity to believe in hope as a virtue. (p. 40)

This Greek critique of hope has all but been forgotten. False hope is especially damaging; hope, when it is little more than consolation, is meaningless. False hope is not speaking truth, it is false. However, to critique hope does not mean sliding down the slippery slope of nihilism. Nihilism leads to barbarism.

Two days after 9/11 commentators began the nonsense- talk of "the healing must begin"; this blather was more than an insult to those left behind; it was an insult to the memory of those who perished. Americans—especially—are uncomfortable with being uncomfortable. The position that false hope is harmful makes many uncomfortable. What hope is there after a tragedy like 9/11? That good comes out of evil is yet another trite expression that is meaningless, for good does not come out of evil, nothing comes out of evil, nothing is learned from suffering, no lessons are at hand. Evil begets more evil.

Although Thomas Merton and Nietzsche could not be more different, in some ways their writings coincide. Merton's theology was not sentimental; Merton did not gloss over harsh realities. Likewise, Nietzsche, ever the harsh critic—of everything—never glossed over anything. Merton continually questioned and countered the status quo. So too did Nietzsche.

Merton argued that faith means struggle and confronting "crisis" (1981, p. 107); that faith, in fact, is "crisis," that theology is "crisis." Merton (1981) argued that

> Christian mysticism is born of theological crisis. This theological crisis is precipitated by the very nature of faith... It "sees" God but only in darkness, *per speculum, in aenigmate*. To see in darkness is not to see. To understand in an enigma is not to understand but to be perplexed. (p. 107).

Recall, I began this book citing Merton: that theology is born of "crisis" and that this book was born of crisis. Some work writing to work through scientific problems; others work writing as a work of mourning. This book is a testament to the work of mourning and Merton is one of the most profound theologians on the work of mourning beside St. John of the Cross. Darkness makes most uncomfortable, but St. John of the Cross insists that it is in that darkness that the soul finds its work. Chaplaincy is certainly the work of mourning, it is a calling through a looking glass darkly, as St. Paul put it.

The Latin phrase *"speculum, in aenigmate"* loosely translates as through a glass darkly. Jewish mysticism—in the Kabbalah—also draws on a metaphor of glass, albeit in a different way to describe the work necessary in living a life. The Kabbalah describes life as broken shards of glass as a metaphor for the brokenness of humanity. Human beings live broken lives; human beings are those broken shards of glass. The task at hand is to pick up the pieces of broken shards of glass; to pick up the pieces of broken lives, not so as to make them happy lives, but so as to make life soulful and to help those continue-on when they cannot. Theology begins in the places where no one wants to look—through that looking-glass darkly. Theology is not, nor should it be a pointing toward paradise. I think Dante got it wrong. He begins his work in the Inferno: All ye who enter here lose hope. His is a traditional Christian narrative of transcendence toward paradise. Perhaps Dante should have remained where he began: in despair, without hope. But, for many Christians—including Kierkegaard—despair is considered a sin. It is ironic the Kierkegaard comes around to that position in his writings because he seems to also emphasize the difficulties and sufferings, the struggles and tribulations, the sacrifices one must make to be a disciple of Christ. But he cannot seem to unlink himself from the progress narrative that one must work through sin to transcendence toward the light. And yet, most of his writings are not about what is light, but through the looking glass darkly.

Merton (1981) points out that for St. John of the Cross "the powers of the soul must be ordered and controlled by reason" (p. 163). The Marxist dialectic can be of use here. Thinking dialectically—a form of "ordered" and "controlled reason" Adorno (1966/2007; 2008)—avoids the problems of reification. Reification is hardened ideology. Rigid ideologies do not help one move through the world; in fact, they are the root cause of authoritarianism(s). Reification of any kind, reification of identity as Robert Musil (1996a; 1996b) writes about in *The Man Without Qualities*, can become rather dangerous.

The Man Without Qualities is a story of the importance of equivocation; an idea that runs counter to Enlightenment philosophy, especially Descartes' stress on certainty and indubitable principles. To equivocate means to trip over oneself; to embrace, in fact, uncertainty and doubt. Although Descartes began his philosophical meditations with doubt, he ends his work arguing that the path to Enlightenment is certainty, and the reification of identity. I think therefore I am (the *Cogito Ergo Sum*) is an example of the reification of identity. But how can one be so sure of anything?

Unlike Descartes, Musil's man *without* qualities does not know who he is, he is unsure of himself. Musil argues it is better to be unsure of oneself than to be too sure, not only of one's identity, but also to not be too sure about one's identity in relation to state or nation, country. What does it mean to be a patriot? We know today—after the January 6th insurrection at the United States Capitol—how the word patriotism can be misused in the service of authoritarianism. Reification of identity is directly related to reification of national identity. Patriotism—a word that is used in the service of violence, or as a validation of White Nationalism—demands critique. Unfortunately, the word patriotism has been co-opted by white nationalists and Neo-Nazis in the name of ethnic cleansing and racism. Rigid identity-politics like white nationalism and Neo-Nazism are exactly what Musil feared. He saw what was happening in his native Austria, even before Hitler occupied Austria. Anti-Semitism in Austria was virulent as it was in many European countries. Today, Anti-Semitism is on the rise not only in Europe but also in the United States. White nationalism, patriotism and extremism have created the perfect storm for the arrival of a newly formed storm trooper. But today storm troopers are dressed in suits and ties and line the halls of congress. We live in very dangerous times, indeed. Musil's writings are still relevant today.

Musil argued that it is better to not adhere to rigid identities, to be a man without qualities is to be a man who equivocates, deliberates: to be a man who is unsure of himself. Deliberation and equivocation are ways to avoid falling into the traps of totalitarianism. Like Musil, Merton felt that embracing—rather than eschewing doubt—drove his life's work and his writing. Living in a state of doubt means embracing an uncomfortable sense of restlessness. It is said that Augustine was a restless soul. It was Augustine's (2008) restlessness that led to the writing of his *Confessions*, one of the most important books in the Christian literature.

Contemplation and Action

Thomas Merton (1981), drawing on St. Gregory of Nyssa, states that the contemplative must become aware of

> Invisible realities which the intellect alone can apprehend. And that is what we have been talking about as *theoria* –and intellectual form of contemplation. This darkening [in the process of thinking theoretically]… is like a cloud in which the soul becomes accustomed to traveling blind. (p. 51)

From a phenomenological perspective it is interesting to note that Maurice Merleau-Ponty (1968) took a similar position in *The Visible and the Invisible*. The body—in a sense—travels blindly in a world of invisibles. There is much to the world that we do not understand; there are mysteries that we cannot see. What we see gets obscured by what we do not see. Merleau-Ponty (1968) compares this problem to Augustine's writings on time. "What Saint Augustine said of time— that it is perfectly familiar to each, but that none of us can explain it to the others must be said of the world" (p. 3). Like the strangeness of time, the world—that which is made up of the visible and invisible— remains strange. One can describe one's experiences, one can draw upon the faculties of reason to attempt to understand the world but still, the world's ineffability remains.

It was James Macdonald (1995) who said that *Theory is a Prayerful Act*. Curriculum theory is not literally prayer, of course. But curriculum theory—as a field unique to the discipline of education—is not afraid to venture into the prayerful, soulful, poetic and ineffable questions about suffering and lived experience. Like the work of Thomas Merton, curriculum theory flies in the in the face of sentimentality; curriculum theory flies in the face of that which is consoling and comfortable. Curriculum theory is a risk-taking field: working on the edges of thought, pressing the boundaries of thought to their edges is risky in an academic culture that is averse to new ways of thinking. Education as a discipline— in particular—is especially reactionary, as it is wedded to what Derrida called vulgar empiricism, with few exceptions.

The Lure of the Transcendent—as Dwyane Huebner (1999) put it—is the lure of the ineffable. Huebner pushed boundaries of thought and was one of the earliest curriculum theorists to insist on the importance of reading broadly outside of the narrow parameters of teaching and learning. In fact, Huebner was highly critical of the term learning because he said it foreclosed on the adventure of education, it foreclosed on free exploration of knowledge outside the narrow confines of the schoolhouse.

Edward Said (1996)—who pushed the boundaries of thought in the realm of postcolonial scholarship—insisted that the intellectual must be "embarrassing and unpleasant" (p. 12). Nietzsche's (2008) "hammer" (p. 3) that Gadfly—as Socrates once put it—irritates, stirs up trouble, throwing the mediocre off guard. Curriculum theorists, too, like Huebner, for example, had little patience for the mediocre; he pushed his students beyond the bounds of the thinkable. He encouraged his students to read everything from theology to philosophy, from literature to the social sciences. Huebner (1999) stated that "My last year in the university was spent in the library and in a seminar with Hans Gerth in advanced social psychology. [He read] Talcott Parsons, Donald Hebbs, Sussanne Langer, Ernst Cassier and Bertrand Russell.... I found myself turning to the mystics of the East and the West including Meister Eckhart.... Marcel, Merleau-Ponty, Jaspers, Sartre" (p. 448). Huebner opened the door for many of us in curriculum studies to do the kind of work that we do. Colleges of education, however, still for the most part are stuck in vulgar empiricism, psychometrics and statistics. Of course there are uses for empiricism, psychometrics and statistics; however, reading more broadly—as did Huebner opens the pathway to the ineffable in education, something educationists—still—fear, or abhor as useless knowledge. Philosophers of education are more open to new ways of thinking and to reading broadly outside of the narrow confines of the schoolhouse.

Thomas Merton and Political Engagement

As Edward Said might have put it, Merton became an "embarrassing and unpleasant" (1996, p. 12) problem for the Catholic Church. For decades the story about Merton's death was that he died in a tragic accident. The Church reported that while Merton was in a bathtub, he accidentally got electrocuted. However, this story has come under scrutiny. Hugh Turley and David Martin (2018) argue—in their controversial book—that Merton was murdered by the CIA because he was seen as a threat to national security. Merton spoke against the Vietnam War.

Merton was a well-known writer and public figure. As Foucault (2008) put it, there is a price to pay for truth-telling; speaking truth to power has consequences. Perhaps the truth about Merton's death will never be known, but Turley and Martin (2018) make a convincing case that Merton's death was not an accident.

Merton emphasized throughout his work that theory and activism needed to fit hand-in-glove. Merton (2007) claimed:

> Wisdom is not only speculative, but also practical: that is to say, it is "lived." And unless one "lives" it, one cannot "have" it. It is not only speculative but creative. It is expressed in living signs and symbols. It proceeds, then, not merely from knowledge about ultimate values, but from an actual possession and awareness of these values as incorporated into one's own existence. (p. 69)

Merton suggests, then, that wisdom is a lived-wisdom. It is not enough to be a contemplative. Merton was a social activist. He felt that he needed to counter what he saw was wrong with a government who fought an unjust war. Vietnam was a catastrophe. Merton was outspoken against this catastrophe. Those who threaten the powerful sometimes pay with their lives. Nietzsche's (2017) *Will to Power* speaks to the problems of might makes right. The United States government has had a long history of regime change—a euphemism for might makes right.

There have been theologians before Thomas Merton who were also activists and died fighting for the rights of oppressed peoples throughout Europe and the Americas. Most notably in the Christian tradition, the Confessing Church—of which Dietrich Bonhoeffer was a member—fought against Hitler's regime. Bonhoeffer's plot to murder Hitler was foiled; Bonhoeffer died at the hands of the Nazis. Romero, the Catholic Priest, was murdered for his missionary work in El Salvador: he, along with nuns were gunned down. The film *Romero* (1989) depicts Oscar Romero's struggles. He was feared by those who wielded power in El Salvador. Liberation theology—after Romero's death—died with him. There have been attempts to resuscitate liberation theology but there are many who critique missionary movements like liberation theology because one of their aims is—in fact—colonization.

Merton (2007), unlike Romero, was not a liberation theologian. He was a Trappist Monk. Merton was a writer, not a revolutionary. Unlike most Trappist monks—who are contemplatives—and not political activists or writers, Merton (2007) argues that "contemplatives... [should be] in the world of art, letters, education, and even politics" (pp. 87-88). Although many churches claim that they are apolitical, the fact of the matter is that religion is inherently political.

Contemplation does not mean removal from the world of politics. In fact, it might, ironically, allow for deeper engagement in the world. Distance from the world—paradoxically—can give one insight into the world. Being too close to things can blind one from what is going on in the world.

Moreover, one does not literally have to march on the front lines to do social activism. William Pinar (2009) makes this point clear in his writings, especially in his work on cosmopolitanism. Pinar writes about the controversial film maker Pier Paolo Pasolini and states that he engaged in political activism through artistry, being a "poet, playwright, and theoretician, always an outsider.... the legendary filmmaker understood his civic commitment as subjective expression of private passion" (p. x). Film, in other words, can become a form of social activism. Pasolini certainly made strong political statements—through film—that rattled those in Italy who wielded power. In fact, many of his films were banned in Italy. Films can have a powerful impact on peoples' view on the world. Films can change people. Like film, books can change people. Marx (1978) stated in his *Theses on Feuerbach*: "The philosophers have only *interpreted* [italics in the original] the world, in various ways; the point, however, is to *change* [italics in the original] it" (p. 145). In many ways, Merton attempted to interpret and change the world.

Merton has much in common with the Italian Marxist Antonio Gramsci, who was imprisoned for his political views. Gramsci wrote against the rising tide of Fascism in Italy, when Mussolini wielded power. Gramsci landed in a Fascist prison, which so weakened him that he died shortly after his release. 2,000 pages of his writings were smuggled out of his jail cell and that is why today we have what is now called Gramsci's *Prison Notebooks* (see, Quintin Hoare & Geoffrey Nowell Smith, 1971). Gramsci's writings have had a long lasting and profound effect on critical theory, activism, and Marxist critique. Gramsci's (1971) insights into Italian Fascism focus on the ways in which power works in authoritarian societies. Gramsci's is a cautionary tale. The United States—as well as many other nations around the globe—is slipping into dictatorship. Gramsci's work still resonates today.

Gramsci and Thomas Merton are still both read to this day. Merton's autobiography—*The Seven Storey Mountain*—has been compared to St. Augustine's (1961) *Confessions*. When *Seven Storey Mountain* was initially published it sold millions of copies world-wide. Merton believed that the life of the writer cannot be—or should not be—separated from what it is that he writes. That is, Merton suggested that philosopher should live a philosophical life; a poet should live a poetic life. Merton (2007) was a theologian who certainly lived a theological life. Merton (2007) states:

> The true philosopher and the true poet become what they are when they "go beyond" philosophy and poetry, and cease to "be philosophers" or to "be poets." It is at that point that their whole lives become philosophy and poetry—in other words, there is no longer any philosophy and or any poetry separable from the unity of their existence. (p. 27)

Academic philosophers are not necessarily what Merton calls "true" philosophers. Not all philosophers live as philosophers. Many academics get bogged down in bureaucracy and forget their calling. The institution of the university is a Kafkaesque world. The university—in many ways—prevents philosophers from living-out their calling because they get so bogged down in administrivia. But Derrida argues that philosophers can fulfill their calling despite these problems. Derrida suggests that philosophers must be housed inside of the university in order to change it. Although the institution of the university is highly problematic, philosophers need a place to work. The work of deconstruction goes hand-in-glove with the philosopher who critiques the very foundation of the institution that houses him. However, there are those who cannot be housed in universities for one reason or another. Walter Benjamin could never land a position in a Germanic university, for one reason or another. He did his work despite the university. In fact, he was quite critical of the German university for its rigidity and conservatism. Then there are those who do not have formal educational training but are street intellectuals; these are the bohemians who do their work, say, at European coffeehouses. In Austria—even today—coffeehouses are places where poets, writers, philosophers meet to discuss intellectual work, many of the coffeehouse intellectuals are not affiliated with universities and do not have academic or formal training. The tradition of the European coffeehouse is the place where one might find what Gramsci called the organic intellectual, the intellectual who does not have formal institutional training. Gramsci's (2000) "organic" (p. 309) intellectuals born of the street.

Although Walter Benjamin was not an "organic" intellectual—because he had formal university training—some suggest that he was better off not being installed in a German university because it either would have broken him—spiritually—-or prevented him from writing the things that he did. His writings fall outside of the frame of traditional academic philosophy. Nobody understood what he was doing; his writings were so far ahead of his time. German universities have been known to be notoriously elitist and conservative. Of course, anti-Semitism was also part of the reason Benjamin could not find a home in Germanic universities; they were not exactly places that were open to Jewish intellectuals, especially in the 1930s and even earlier.

Erving Goffman (1961) pointed out that the "total institution's" function is to break people. Mental institutions, prisons, the military, law school serve as "total institutions" where the purpose of that institution is to break you, to break your will. Broken spirits have a difficult time staying true to their professorial calling. The very place that is supposed to foster intellectual life, breaks it. That Walter Benjamin never landed an academic position perhaps worked in his favor. Some suggest that Walter Benjamin could never have produced the kind of intellectual work that he did had he landed an academic position.

Michel Serres (1998) comments that the university a battleground; its sole function is to kill the mind. Serres was highly critical of university culture and compared university politics to warfare.

Like university culture, the monastic life comes with its own problems as well. It too serves as a "total institution." (Goffman, 1961). The monastic life is not dissimilar to the military. Monastic life is one of discipline and regimentation. Merton's situation might have been unique, however because he seemed to have freedoms that other Trappist monks do not. However, it is not clear whether Merton ever felt at home in the monastery. He seemed troubled, tormented, in fact, by his double life as writer and Trappist monk. Yet, somehow he managed to make his situation workable.

Merton thought of himself not only as theologian, but as a philosopher-poet. In *Echoing Silence* Merton (2007) states that poetry can be "revolutionary" (p. 99). Merton felt that poetry could serve as a call to action; and, indeed, he felt that poetry was a form of activism in-and-of-itself. Merton (2007) states

> The poets have much to say and do: they have the same mission as the prophets in the technical world. They have to be the consciousness of the revolutionary man because they have the keys to the subconscious.... But governments are full of poet-killers and of anti-poets with machines to fabricate only death and nothing more. Then, the future of poetry depends upon their freedom, the freedom of conscience and creation. (p. 99)

Merton (2007) like other poets of his generation—Allen Ginsburg, Lawrence Ferlinghetti, Kenneth Patchen—also engaged in poetry-as-activism. They worked against the power of the "poet-killers." They were outspoken against the Vietnam war, as was Merton.

State run universities are under the thumb of the government. State universities can also become "poet-killers" (p. 99). For philosophers and poets, theologians and educationists, generally speaking, universities can become battlegrounds, as Serres (1998) pointed out. This is why Derrida (1992) wrote—in *Logomachia: The Conflict of the Faculties*— that it would be in the best interest of intellectuals to re-invent the university. Where can intellectuals do their work in peace? Derrida suggested that intellectuals might not be better off working under the thumb of administrators. Adorno (2008) pointed out that a highly administered culture is dangerous. This, too, was Kafka's (1998) worry. *The* Castle—like the university—houses bureaucracies, within bureaucracies, within bureaucracies. The point of a bureaucracy is to destroy the human spirit—Kafka stressed. The university-as-castle-as bureaucracy is a militarized zone.

Leaving graduate school with diploma-in-hand does not prepare one for what is to come in the castle that is the university— the "poet-kill[ing]" (Merton, 2007, p. 27) bureaucracy. Hours and hours of wasted time engaging in meaningless committee work serves no real purpose. Faculty governance is non-existent, but faculty is called to govern. Tenure—something taken-for-granted by faculty—is now under erasure in Republican held strongholds in the United States. Still, faculty must sit on tenure committees, even though tenure does not exist. Faculty handbooks tout academic freedom, but university professors are summarily fired for speaking up against the lack of vaccine mandates. Although professors operate under the assumption that due process is part of any termination, due process no longer exists in right-to-work states where one can be fired without cause. A right-to-work state means that the state has the right to fire anyone without cause. These are Kafkaesque realities. How do scholars survive the battlefield that is the university? Serres worried that they do not. In fact, Serres said before he died that the future of the humanities—especially—is no-future at all. Neo-liberal universities are killing the humanities, for the humanities, officials say, are useless. The only useful disciplines—conservatives claim—are those that are tied directly to the market. The useless disciplines—without utilitarian function—have no place in the university. The useless disciplines of philosophy, theology, the arts and the humanities are on the chopping blocks at many universities.

The university—although claiming a non for-profit status—functions as if it is for-profit, but no one knows where those profits go. How is it that a football coach makes more money than most university presidents? Where does that money come from? Profits made from sporting events? Where does that money go? Certainly not to faculty members. Intellectuals installed in universities and in schools are treated as little more than cannon fodder—as the pandemic rages on. Putting professors and teachers in dangerous situations—classrooms that are unventilated, over crowded with students who have covid or are forced back to school before they are well—is unconscionable. And yet the work of the university continues unabated as faculty are forced to serve on meaningless tenure committees when tenure no longer exists. Faculty committees are under the false assumption that there is faculty governance, but university senate committees are not run by faculty members, they are run and controlled by administrators. Even if faculty members speak at senate meetings, their words fall on deaf ears. The university mirrors the larger cultural disaster that is United States democracy. We are on the brink of losing our democracy.

Merton (2007) calls "unnatural, frantic, anxious work [that work that is] done under pressure of greed or fear" (p. 76). This anxious, tedious, ridiculous and petty, meaningless "frantic" culture of university service work becomes increasingly more busy, tedious, more bureaucratic, more Kafkaesque (1998). Gatekeepers before the law—who prevent intellectuals from doing their work—are guarded by more and more (administrative) gatekeepers, keeping out unwanted peoples and dangerous knowledges.

Nietzsche (2004) writes about what he saw as the most basic problem in Germanic universities in the late 19th century as "[t]wo opposing streams, [both colliding to] equally ruinous [ends]" (p. 17). Nietzsche (2004) states "one stream of university culture fostered [*Bildung*] [which Nietzsche would later critique for its dangerous apolitical nature] and on the other side... the diminution and the weakening of the same" (p. 17) through technocratic practical training. But perhaps for Nietzsche, the most dangerous aspect of what he saw as the demise of Germanic universities was that which "subordinate[s] itself serving another form of life, namely that of the state" (p. 17). State run universities are especially troublesome because dictatorial policies are too easily mandated. Nietzsche anticipated the German university catastrophe as Hitler installed his own (mostly incompetent) professors, getting rid of Jewish professors and students, cleansing libraries of books written by Jewish intellectuals. Heidegger, the Rector of Freiburg University, fell in line with Hitler's Final Solution. Heidegger has no problem firing Jewish professors, getting rid of Jewish students and cleansing the library of Jewish books. This still shocks philosophers who are wedded to Heidegger's work; philosophers still do not know what to do with Heidegger's legacy and his intellectual contributions. Can one separate the life of the man Heidegger—who was a Nazi—and the work of the philosopher (i.e., Heidegger's

(1962) *Being and Time*)—one of the most important philosophical texts written in the 20th century.

Drawing on Kant's (1979) *Conflict of the Faculties,* Derrida (1992), in *Logomachia,* points out that Kant "recognize[d] a conflict at the universities very interior" (p. 13). Derrida (1992) remarks that Kant felt that what was "dangerous" were "organization[s] of specialized scholars into academies or societies. These 'workshops' do not belong to the university" (p. 13). Derrida (1992) points out that currently "there can be very serious competition and border-conflicts between non-university centers of research and university faculties claiming at once to be doing research" (p. 14). Derrida (1992) reports in Europe "the state no longer entrust[s] certain investigations to a university that cannot accept the structures or control of the techno-political stakes" (p. 14). Most disturbingly, Derrida (1992) points out that "in certain Eastern [European] countries, the university is totally confined to the pursuit of reproducible teaching. The state deprives it of the right to do research, reserved for academies without teachers" (p. 14). "Reproducible teaching"—based on a factory model—haunts public schools and universities in the United States as well. In the United States—in alignment with reactionary state policies—"reproducible teaching" is becoming more and more common. To standardize not only teaching but the knowledges that are taught turns the curriculum into a Ford Factory. Intellectual freedom is disappearing from the academy as reactionary policies—like "reproducible teaching" or "teaching to the test" or the erasure of the horrors of history from the curriculum get mandated. Whitewashing curriculum—that the Civil War was, in fact, a war of aggression, that slavery was not so bad for the slaves because at least they had food and housing, that the recent disaster that was the January 6th insurrection at the United States Capitol will not be allowed to be taught in public schools, that anything that makes white people "uncomfortable" in the classroom can no longer be taught. What is happening in public schools around the country is trickling up to state run universities as well. What is next? Who is next? Book burnings on campuses are allowed, for they are little more than freedom of speech; spouting hate in the classroom is little more than freedom of speech. And it is one's freedom not to get vaccinated: my body, my choice; but it is the Other's problem—so reactionaries say—if the unvaccinated infect the vulnerable with covid. Yet when it comes to the "rights of the unborn" it is not a woman's choice to control her own body. It is not her body, her choice when abortion is outlawed. Roe v. Wade was considered sacrosanct, until the supreme court thought otherwise. What was once considered settled law, is now unsettled law. How do left-leaning intellectual survive in reactionary times? Censorship is everywhere on university campuses, especially those run by reactionary governors. Speaking truth to power is a risky endeavor, even when academic freedom is (falsely) touted.

Derrida (1992) says that Kant noted that "the technical administration of knowledge" meant that professors would be "subject[ed] by law, to the control of the faculties, 'to the censorship of the faculties', as Kant literally says" (p. 17). Kant stated that censorship was the "most odious tyranny" (cited in Derrida, 1992, p. 17). Kant and Nietzsche both noted the demise of academic freedom even in universities in the 18th and 19th centuries.

It seems ironic that Thomas Merton—a Trappist monk cloistered in the Abbey of Gethsemani in Kentucky—had more intellectual freedom than most intellectuals housed in universities. John Henry Newman (1852)—who wrote *The Idea of the University*—stated that the great philosophers "shunned the lecture room and the public school. Pythagoras... lived for a time in a cave. Thales... lived unmarried and in private... refused the invitations of princes. Plato withdrew from Athens to the groves of the Academus" (p. 10). Interestingly, Michel Serres once said that scholars would be much better off spending time at retreats than attending academic conferences. The idle chatter and posturing that goes on at academic conferences is hardly intellectual work.

I think that many are drawn to Merton's struggles because in his autobiography he paints himself as one who does *not* know what he is doing. His doubt and torment about his need to write while his vows of silence as a Trappist monk seemed at loggerheads. Merton appeals to many who are also plagued by doubt and confusion in their own lives.

Merton lived a theology of the *via negativa*; he lived a theological life on the edge of being, if you will. Merton claimed that the seeming absence of God was, in actuality, a sign of grace. Why hast thou forsaken me? Is this God's grace? Kierkegaard would say yes. The suffering servant—the Christ—endured absence, silence, nothingness.

Kathleen Deignan (2007) comments that Merton's "journals are replete with confessions of exhaustion" (p. 33). This, indeed, is what Dietrich Bonhoeffer (1937/1995) called *The Cost of Discipleship*. Like Merton, Bonhoeffer engaged in writing and political activism. Bonhoeffer was murdered by the Nazis, as his plot to kill Hitler was foiled, as was mentioned earlier. Bonhoeffer paid the *cost of discipleship* with his life. Like Bonhoeffer, Merton (1998) states emphatically that

> No matter what religious Order a man enters, whether its Rule be easy or strict in itself does not much matter.; if his vocation is to be really fruitful it must cost him

something, and must be a real sacrifice. It must be a cross, a true renunciation of natural goods, even of the highest natural goods. (p. 319)

Taking vows of monasticism is not unlike taking vows of the professoriate. The task of the intellectual is a serious one. Yet, there are—in actuality— few *intellectuals* housed in universities. Petty bureaucrats—-as Kant, Nietzsche and Kafka knew all too well—fill the halls of academe, selling out to the state, playing a kind of *Glass Bead Game*—as Herman Hesse (1943/1990) put it—to please administrators. Few academics take seriously the cost of (intellectual) discipleship. A true intellectual speaks truth to power; a true intellectual sacrifices time, investing in the very labor necessary for intellectual discovery. Most do not realize the time that true intellectuals invest in their work. Scholarship is a demanding task; the art of writing and thinking, teaching and mentoring involves a serious commitment to one's calling. The true intellectual devotes a lifetime to thought and writing, teaching and mentoring.

Merton (2007) claims

No writing on the solitary, meditative dimensions of life can say anything that has not already been said better by the wind in the pine trees.... But what can the wind say where there is no hearer? There is then a deeper silence: the silence in which the hearer is No-hearer. That deeper silence must be heard before one can speak truly of solitude. (p. 55)

Merton compares himself to Thoreau and, in fact, states that it was at the monastery where he read *Walden* (2021). For Thoreau, nature was infused with the divine; the silence of nature speaks only when one can hear—in a profound way—what it is that the wind is saying, what the waters of a river are asking of us. Merton felt that the "wind in the pine trees" shed more wisdom than the anxious business of everyday life. Still, Merton was not at peace, even as he took refuge in nature. He found a "deeper silence" (2007, p. 55) in the pine trees, and yet, like Augustine, Merton was forever restless.

Merton's continual theological crisis, his perpetual restlessness and uncertainty can serve as a foundationless foundation, a curriculum without a curricula, if you will. A curriculum without a curriculum is an education without foreclosure, an education on the edge. There is no standardized, pre-fabricated curriculum for living through a pandemic, for instance. This horror we are living through is foundationless; the unprecedented demands an unprecedented curricula, one without borders, boundaries, or limits. Standardized and pre-fabricated curricula taught in formal institutions have not prepared us for the covid-19 catastrophe that is unfolding before us.

As Merton merged with the theology of the *via negativa*, so, too, might intellectuals merge with *via negativa* of the pandemic. Like the life of the intellectual, the life of the hospital chaplain is one of *walking with* the *via negativa, walking through* the *via negativa*. The unbearable theological crisis at hand means facing squarely continual doubt and uncertainty about everything, about life, death and the larger question of why. Why now? Why us? Why did that child have to die? Who answers? Where are the answers? There are no answers. We are left in the darkness of the valley of the shadow of death; the death of the Other, the death of our own spirits.

This exhaustion—about which Merton pondered in the context of his own life struggles—is beyond signification. Jean-Luc Nancy (1996) eloquently states: "There is neither resurrection nor assumption. There is more and less than a negotiation or a philosophy of death. There is neither abyss, nor ecstasy, nor salvation" (p. 65). Nancy (1996) lived on the edge of life and death; he knew only too well that life in the face of death overwhelms to the point of exhaustion. Nancy—who had a heart transplant—who hovered on the "threshold" as he puts it of death for decades—knew only too well, what it meant to live in a precarious state. Can we build community in this time of the pandemic? Or is community—yet—another modernist notion that collapses under the weight of trauma?

As Nancy (1991) struggled with the notion of community—in his remarkable book *The Inoperative Community*, it seems that he at once wants to resurrect the notion of community but simultaneously realizes that community is no longer a viable concept in the traditional sense of the word. Nancy surmises that the traditional notion of community is—at the end of the day—inoperative. Nancy (1991), in the context of how to frame the idea of community, states

> It is as though Bataille, despite the constancy of his concern and intentions, was led nonetheless to endure the extremity of the distressed world in which he lived—this world at war, torn apart by an atrocious negation of community and a mortal conflagration of ecstasy. In this severe affliction he no longer saw any face, any schema, or even any simple point of reference for community, now that the figures of religious or mystical communities belonged to the past. (p. 22)

It would seem that community would be the most important thing to which we might hold onto during these days of the pandemic. But in the face of so much trauma, community—as an idea—has vanished. In a Hobbesian world—a dog-eat-dog, war-against-all world where covid has ignited more violence than can be contained –community is no longer. Divisions, schisms, battles, insurrections, bloodshed—violence-writ-large has demonstrated that the idea of community is a mere myth. The absolute breakdown of community has become more and more pronounced, even at the death bed. Death—especially during the pandemic—brings out the worst in families. Oedipal dramas and struggles that perhaps were dormant prior to covid—have come to the fore. Family members who attempt to cope with death cannot. Brother fights with brother. Sister fights with sister. And sometimes brothers and sisters kill one another. Gun violence has skyrocketed since the onset of covid. Rage—the most primary emotion—is the only way some can deal with the pandemic. Chaplains—sometimes—are also a target of rage—for they represent the angel of death, bearing bad news.

Nancy (1991) was a deeply religious person. How one holds onto faith until the end is a mystery, as is faith, I suppose. Nancy (1991) says, "We alone are lost" (p. 11). We are all lost in the midst of the chaos of a pandemic.

The unvaccinated continue in strangely held beliefs that scientists do not know anything. The unvaccinated believe that vaccines are little more than poison, or hocus pocus. The sad truth is that the majority of people dying today of covid are the unvaccinated. Those who are vaccinated—the medical staff especially— conceal their own feelings of resentment against the unvaccinated—the very people they are taking care of. The unvaccinated are putting everyone at risk, including their own children.

Covid is contaminating the very air that we breathe. Derrida (2005) remarks

> Contamination then becomes what it is not; it disidentifies itself. It disidentifies everything even before it disidentifies *itself*. (italics in the original] It disappropriates itself, it attains what it should never signify, namely an interruption of relations and the ex-propriety of the proper. (p. 75)

Whether one has been contaminated by the very air that sustains life, whether it is the Other who has been contaminated—Derrida rightly suggests that the contaminated—in this case by covid-19—"signifies" what it should not: "an interruption of relations" (p. 75) between the self and the Other. This is what Derrida means by the "ex-propriety of the proper."

Death and theological resentments, rage against the machine of this horrific virus, will not go silently into that good night. "We alone are lost" (Nancy, 1991, p. 11) and yet all of us are lost. The very foundations of all of our institutions have been thrown into question and chaos. Universities, hospitals, schools, prisons—"We alone are lost"—and yet we are all lost. The communities around which these institutions were once built are, as Nancy would say "shattered" (p. 82). The shattering of peoples' lives in the face of covid is everywhere around us. In the classroom, in the hospital, in the prison.

This shattering and fear that the Other might be contagious—has wrecked any sense of communing together. At the bottom, everyone is afraid of everyone else. This fear drives us apart, drives us mad. Who has covid? Who tested positive? Who in this class is carrying covid? Where is the contact tracing? There is no contact tracing. The visible and the invisible—what is more dangerous? This phrase is No longer poetic—as Merleau-Ponty once coined it. The invisible (virus) shatters any sense of stability we might have once had. Time is out of joint, as Shakespeare once said. Nothing is right with the world. Education-writ-large has utterly failed us. Our theologies make little sense. Philosophy cannot contain this catastrophe.

We have no stories upon which to base our experience. There are neither philosophies nor theologies that serve as foundations in this foundationless mess we are in. And yet we write what we know because that is all we have. Indeed, "We alone are lost" (Nancy, 1991. P. 11). Yet, Nancy also suggests that it is the "inscription" (p. 80), the writing, the archivization—as Derrida might put it—that sustains us, at least for a while. What the "inscription" of education does teach, however, is that whatever it is that we confront—and in this case, we confront a terrible pandemic—we have our texts, we have our disciplines, we have the arts, cinema, painting, music and so forth, that might sustain us for a little while. Merton, so conflicted by the "inscription"—his need to write, his call to write—lived the paradox of a life inscribed by contradictions. His vow of silence contradicted his need to write. We live a time of paradox, in a terrible paradox indeed. The very air that sustains us can also kill.

5

The Unbearable Stories of Terry Tempest Williams, Joan Didion and Derrick Jensen

Covid-19 rages on. Year three into the pandemic and things have gotten worse. The delta and lambda variants have been joined by omicron, and deltacron, the flu and delta variant have also combined. In the United States there is no national mandate for vaccines. Children are being admitted to the hospitals at alarming rates; some are even on ventilators. Hospital staff is thinning as omicron is highly contagious and many health care workers are out sick. There seems no end to this global nightmare. We are still too close to this historical catastrophe to make much sense of the stories that we hear. It will take decades to begin to unpack what has happened.

Putting Concepts to Work: Unbearable Stories

Generally speaking, the highly conceptual chapters in this book had to be hammered out—as Nietzsche would put it— in order to then put concepts to work in the sense that Adorno (1966/2007) called for when writing his incredible work titled *Negative Dialectics*. Adorno (2008) suggests that the problem with concepts is that they tend to get "reified" (p. 24). Adorno (2008) explains that "a reified consciousness... bring[s] all the concepts in the world to a standstill simultaneously and... fetishize[s] them" (p. 24). This suggests that concepts or Ideologies—like vulgar interpretations of Marxism or psychoanalysis, for example— become little more than "headlines in advertisements" (Adorno, 2008, p. 24)—if they are used over and over again as jargon or catch-phrases. Vulgar Marxism reduces the complexities of Marxist ideas to one or two over-arching principles, like capital or alienated labor. Marxism reduced to capital and/or alienated labor puts under erasure the complexities of Marx's ideas. There is far more to Marx than capital and/or alienated labor. The same could be said of psychoanalysis—as it is sometimes reduced to pathology, or defense mechanisms. Psychoanalysis is far more complicated than pathology and/or defense mechanisms. In order to avoid reification and simplification of ideas, Adorno suggests that concepts and ideas demand "ceaseless self-renewal" (1966/2007, p. 33).

The more theoretical chapters in this book, say, on Derrida and Serres, for example, lean on concepts that are most amenable to change, to flux, to re-doing and reconceptualizing. The malleability of the major concepts upon which I draw is especially important in the context of putting the concepts to work against the fluid situation of covid-19. Moreover, when applying concepts to unbearable stories there is an even greater difficulty at hand because the very unbearableness of stories—especially around traumatic events—belies concepts. Still, we must have some way of interpreting stories, no matter how unbearable they are; concepts are thus necessary in order to interpret that which is beyond signification—as impossible and contradictory as that might sound.

The conceptual, Adorno suggests, should point to what is non-conceptual, to what Adorno (1966/2007) calls "nonconceptualities" (p. 11). In a way, stories—especially if they are unbearable—do not lend themselves easily to the conceptual. Stories are non-conceptual—that they are not told in the service, say, of philosophy (which is about concept building), but in the service of what needs to be told. But again we need concepts in order to interpret stories. In fact, the more unbearable the stories, the more complicated the concepts must be in order to interpret that which is beyond signification or perhaps even understanding.

In the context of this book and the work I do on the ground, both as a chaplain and as a professor on a university campus are part of the story told here. What I have witnessed—both as a chaplain and professor—have shaped my perspective on this particular historical juncture. Living through a time of pandemic and trying to capture historically what is happening is the impossible task I put to myself. As one person trying to make sense of continual tragedy my story is of course perspectival and affected as a first-person witness who is also part of the trauma. When one writes about the trauma the story that is told is partial and perhaps belies the clinical. Work in the field—the clinical work of being a chaplain—is one thing. But it is altogether different when one tries to tell the story that one sees unfolding. My perspective is just that. One perspective. This is not a clinical account of the pandemic; I am not a scientist and offer no scientific data in the telling of the story. What autobiographic remarks I make throughout the book are perspectival and sometimes perhaps even flawed. But living through a trauma—on this kind of global scale—is something that must be documented from first person(s) accounts. Historians will have a different story to tell after some time passes. But I felt that it was my responsibility to tell the story as I witnessed it from the ground level. Not many have witnessed life from the covid wards: I have. And I also tell the story of someone who has gotten ill from covid, which also gives me a perspective that differs from those who have not gotten ill from this virus. My viewpoint then comes both from my witnessing—on the front lines (both as a chaplain and as a professor)—what is going on, and also from my own experience getting sick from this virus. To tell such a complicated story then—from the ground—demands theoretical work in order to interpret clinical work.

In the hospital my work as a clinical chaplain is very different from my work as a teacher on a university campus. Yet, in both settings, I am dealing with the covid crisis. In both settings (the hospital and the university) and in both roles (as chaplain and as professor) my experiences and thinking about the covid catastrophe continually change as the virus changes. What I have witnessed—especially working in the hospital—cannot be reduced to the conceptual either. the Lives lost to covid-—those lives I have witnessed fading into death—are not reducible to concepts. People are not concepts. Witnessing patients dying is not even amenable to conceptualization on the most existential level. And yet if the stories are to be told, one must have a way to tell the stories; one must have a way to interpret the stories, especially if they are unbearable. Thus, the task at hand is rather difficult because there is a gap between what can be understood and interpreted and what cannot be understood. There is something that is unspeakable about witnessing death. But speak we must. Silence is not the answer.

As a professor on a university campus I see this tragedy getting played out in classrooms in very different ways from my work as a clinical chaplain in a hospital. The frustrations of faculty members who have been thrown into dangerous situations in classrooms with poor ventilation and the lack of mask or vaccine mandates creates tremendous anxiety and fear—not just for faculty but for students as well. State legislatures—in mostly Republican strongholds—refuse to honor faculty demands to work in safer environments. The necessity of having good ventilation in classrooms, the necessity of masks and vaccine mandates, contact tracing and transparency are not being honored in state schools run mostly by conservative legislators. This is not the case in some private universities and private schools around the country. Still, teachers and students—far too often—are put in grave danger because they are forced into unsafe environments.

As a hospital chaplain I have to be present in the face of danger. Chaplains and medical staff are fulfilling an oath to take care of the sick even though our own lives are in danger. We stepped onto covid wards knowing the risks and responsibilities to which we agreed. But school teachers, professors and college students did not take oaths to put their lives in danger. It is the duty of the state and federal government to protect students and teachers, professors and staff.

Living in a time that seems like we are teetering on the edge, never knowing what will come puts to the test the amount of anxiety people can handle. Whether we are theorists or clinicians, at this juncture in history most of us have known someone who has suffered from covid, or who has covid currently, or who has had covid several times, or perhaps most of us know of someone who has died from covid. The stories of covid are yet to be told.

In the meanwhile, we can still learn from stories that have been told—unbearable stories—that have already been archived and well established in the trauma literature. It is important to point out that not that all traumas are the same; nor are traumas experienced in the same ways. No trauma is like another and there are few patterns of similarity in the ways in which traumatic stories get told. However, we can learn from those who have suffered traumas in the past and have told their stories.

Terry Tempest Williams, Joan Didion & Derrick Jensen

This chapter focuses on three very different unbearable stories told by Terry Tempest Williams, Joan Didion and Derrick Jensen. These three stories have been archived and are part of the trauma literature; in fact, they are part of what I call a curriculum of trauma, a curriculum of unbearable stories. These writers represent different traditions, disciplines and ideological persuasions. These catastrophic stories—again—are in no way meant to serve as comparisons, as if to point out patterns or similarities. The point here is to show just the opposite. Here I want to stress how different people from different backgrounds and disciplines and political persuasions write about that which is unbearable. One will find remarkable differences in the telling of these unbearable stories. And it is the differences that I want to focus on.

Those who are now suffering from covid or know others who have died from covid can make use of these stories. These storytellers are companions along life's path; these storytellers are companions in hard times. I found that when I suffered through covid, not once but twice, I found companionship when reading stories of others who had suffered through the unspeakable. These readerly companions did not serve as a balm of Gilead—as it were—but they gave me a sense that I was not alone. Covid isolates people. Before covid, the hospital where I serve as chaplain used to have the following policy: No one dies alone. That policy no longer holds. Covid patients do die alone. And perhaps this is what is most tragic about this illness. Covid wards are isolation wards. Families cannot visit loved ones even during the final moments of life. Covid wards are lonely places.

The concepts that emerge from these unbearable stories in this chapter—i.e. Derridean concepts such as the archive, the trace and difference, or Serres' notions of turbulence, noise, or the clinamen, are useful in that they can be tools of interpretation.

As I emphasized on my work on The Holocaust (Morris, 2001), I am not writing about these unbearable stories in order to teach something, or in order to turn these stories into lessons. There is no pedagogical purpose in writing this book. There is nothing to *learn* from suffering. Suffering just is. Death just is. There is no lesson before dying—as Ernest Gains once put it—-there are no lessons to learn from death. This book is not a pedagogical exercise. I have nothing to teach about watching people die; death teaches nothing. When Socrates was accused of corrupting the youth and was sentenced to death, his advice to his friends was to take care of themselves. It is difficult to take care of ourselves during a time of a global pandemic. Of course, as Serres (1991) points out pandemics have always been around; Ancient Greece and Rome experienced pandemics. Pandemics will always be with us, now and in the future to come.

Pandemics bring pandemonium and death on massive scales. We are seeing that unfold right now, right before our eyes, during our lifetime. Nicolas Diat (2019) sought out monks whom he thought could teach him something about death because they had witnessed so many deaths, living the lives of monastics. Diat (2019) states

> In this desolate world, I had the idea to take the path of the great monasteries in order to discover what the monks might have to teach us about death. Behind cloister walls, they pass their existence in prayer and reflection on the last things.

> I thought their testimony could help people understand suffering, sickness, pain, and the final moments of life. They have known complicated deaths, quick deaths, simple deaths. (p. 13)

Like monastics, chaplains, too, are witnesses to deaths. Yes, I have seen "complicated" deaths, and "quick" deaths. But I have nothing to teach. There are no pedagogical lessons at hand. I know nothing about death. What lessons do we learn from death? None. When I stand with a family of a dying patient, I am there to listen, not to teach. Chaplaincy is a form of negative dialectics—as Adorno might put it. I am not there to tell families anything. I perform a negative theology. I am there—as D. W. Winnicott—might put it—to offer a holding environment. I hold the pain that the families cannot contain. I am nothing more than a container. In my presence (as a chaplain) I offer an absence—of ego. I am a container—an absence of self—for those who are left to speak their sorrows. The sorrows and anguish of those who remain after the death of a loved one are about them, not about me. I am a receptacle—as Plato might have put it in *The Timeaus*. I am present in my absence as a container for those who survive so that they can give testimony to their grief. As Levinas (1985) puts it "Ethical testimony is a revelation which is not a knowledge" (p. 108). Levinas is right to point out ethical testimony—as he calls it—it is not knowledge. But neither do I think that death brings with it "revelation" either. People do not arrive at revelation by speaking their pain. They arrive nowhere; they arrive at a place of utter abandonment. If anything, one might call this a non-revelation; witnessing the death of the Other is the experience of no-thing-ness. Death is nothing. Nothing happens. Nothing. The heart stops beating, the brain stops working. And then silence. Nothing. No revelation is at hand. And it is in that moment of nothingness that we stand together and say nothing to one another. Because, really, there is nothing to say, except perhaps—as Socrates might suggest—take care of yourself. And I am a mere footnote standing in thousands of rooms where patients have died; I am a mere footnote to the anguish families go through witnessing a loved one's death. But the problem with covid is that families are not present at the death of their loved ones. We do have technologies like web-ex that allow for families to see patients through the looking glass darkly as Paul might have put it. But what kind of death is that? To witness someone die through a computer screen, through a glass-enclosed room?

Terry Tempest Williams

Terry Tempest Williams' (2001) *Refuge* is a story of unbearable loss. Although this story is not about covid, what emerges from the story anticipates the kinds of experiences of loss I have witnessed from those who are left behind after losing someone to covid. The idea of refuge for Williams is a complicated one. The very thing that gave her refuge—nature, bird watching, the landscape of the West—became the very thing that killed her mother and most of the women in her family. Her refuge also became her torment. In the 1950s nuclear testing in the deserts of the Utah and elsewhere so totally devastated everything. The nuclear fallout—which the military denied and covered up for many years—killed Williams' family members. All of the women in Williams' family died of cancer.

Michel Serres (1995) has written about why he got out of science. Serres states that while he was in the Navy and learned of Hiroshima and Nagasaki and the sheer disregard of the much of the scientific community about what had occurred, he became outraged, disgusted and lost respect for the discipline of science. Science without ethics is not science: it is barbarism. Serres (1998) states:

> Our generation had an inkling of this day of reckoning, since it saw the dawn of the atomic bomb. Hiroshima was truly the end of one world and the beginning of a new adventure. Science had gained such power that it could virtually destroy the planet. (p. 87)

One would think that after the disgraceful annihilation of the Japanese people, that nuclear power might be reigned in. But it was not. In fact, after the war, nuclear testing continued—mostly in the Western region of the United States; nuclear testing continued in the desert, as if nothing had ever happened.

It is shocking to think that what we learned in school as children seemed so convincing. As an elementary school student I can recall learning that the reason the United States dropped bombs on Japan was to "save lives." School children—still very young—do not have the tools to question what it is that adults teach. Children trust teachers; we were taught that what our government did—at Hiroshima and Nagasaki—was the right thing. This is exactly how school children are mis-educated. Perhaps the teachers believed what they learned; perhaps the social studies texts read in such a way as to support what the government had done without a second thought.

However, decades later, and as Terry Tempest Williams points out, questions began to arise as to the why and the how the ethicality of dropping bombs on innocent civilians was justified by the military and the government. It is quite remarkable that the lies we are told as children stick with us for decades on end. Terry Tempest Williams' story is both a personal and a political one. This is what makes her memoir so incredibly powerful. In fact, she was such a threat to the state legislature of Utah that upon taking her students to a demonstration to protest an ecological atrocity, she was summarily fired from her tenured position at the University of Utah. Questioning politics in the age of reactionary aligned state institutions is a dangerous game, still today.

Williams' (2001) memoir begins with an aporia—as Derrida would put it. This aporia is worth re-iterating. The refuge—the very place that she and her grandmother Mimi used to birdwatch—was the place that became cancerous and deadly; her refuge became a toxic atmosphere that killed all of the women in her family. The toxic land, the toxic environment from continual nuclear testing in the desert of Utah, became the death of countless numbers.

Williams writes about the refuge as a multilayered concept that ties into death and dying, response and responsibility—Derrida might put it. Williams (2001) states:

> When most people had given up on the Refuge, saying the birdswere gone, I was drawn further into its essence. In the same way that when someone is dying many retreat, I chose to stay. (p. 4)

Rachel Carson (1962), the beloved ecologist who wrote one of the most important texts on the destruction of the ecosphere through toxic chemicals—namely DDT, begins her book *Silent Spring* with the disappearance of birds. She states that when the birds go silent, something has gone wrong. Indeed, DDT—when it was legal in the United States—killed not only the birds, but people and other sentient beings. Rachel Carson was excoriated by scientists and the DDT profit-driven industry. Her campaign against DDT finally succeeded, however. DDT was banned in the United States.

Williams (2001) suggests that the birds' *disappearances* from the bird refuge—she and her grandmother Mimi used to visit—serves are as a metaphor for the way in which some people are abandoned when they are dying. Abandonment is a form of disappearance and is surprisingly common when family members become gravely ill; I have witnessed the disappearance and abandonment of gravely ill patients by their family members numerous times (as a hospital chaplain). It is unconscionable to abandon a gravely ill patient who is dying alone from terminal cancer. Husbands abandon wives; wives abandon husbands. Children abandon their parents; parents abandon their children. Covid has created a culture of dying alone: covid wards are places of forced abandonment. No families can visit dying loved ones on covid floors. The best medical staff can do is to offer web ex viewings through glass-enclosed rooms. There is something so impersonal and inhumane about witnessing a loved one die through a computer screen. But this is the only technology that makes the final visitation possible. Still, even with the technology covid patients die alone.

Terry Tempest Williams (2001)—however—did not abandon dying family members. In fact, *Refuge* is the story of Williams' close relationship with her dying mother from the day she was diagnosed with ovarian cancer until the day she died. Terry Tempest Williams *dives into the wreck*—as Adrianne Rich might put it—and is not afraid to confront that which is unbearable.

Williams' story centers mostly on her mother's ovarian cancer and eventual death; this is a gut-wrenching story from beginning to end. Williams' story is, indeed, horrific. Ovarian cancer is not often written about because not many live to tell the tale. And those who are left behind do not often document what they have been through because this is not a narrative of hope; there are usually no winners in the battle against ovarian cancer, unlike some other cancers that people can survive.

Most women who develop ovarian cancer in advanced stages die within five years after diagnosis. There has been little medical progress on ovarian cancer since Williams' mother succumbed to this disease. Most of the research monies for women's cancers go towards breast cancer, not ovarian cancer. By the time most ovarian cancers are detected it is in late stages and it is too late for remission. Ovarian cancer can move from stage one to stage four within one year's time; in most cases women do not experience symptoms. It is often said that ovarian cancer is an invisible killer. Ovarian cancer is stealthy; it moves fast; and it metastasizes, quickly attacking the lungs, the brain, the liver, and the colon. When women do experience symptoms, physicians often miss the signs or dismiss the complaints as mere heartburn or hypochondria. These dismissals are symptoms—as Derrida would put it—of the larger problem of misogyny in the medical community. Tracing misogyny in the medical community is not hard to do; misogyny is rampant in medicine and it has been that way for decades. Derrida (1976) remarks that a "trace... does not let itself be summed up in the simplicity of the present" (p. 66). Misogyny has been deeply historically entrenched not only in medicine, but in the broader culture at large. Freud's word "hysterical" initiated the reification of psycho-somatic illness (beginning with Freud's famous case study on one Dora). Dora's bizarre physiological symptoms like fainting spells and what appeared to be epileptic fits had no basis in physiology. Hysteria then became associated with women's psychological illnesses. However, ovarian cancer is hardly psycho-somatic. It is deadly. And still, to this day ovarian cancer is missed by medical professionals. This is partly why so many women die of ovarian cancer; it goes undetected until it is too late. There are no tests for ovarian cancer, like there are for breast cancer.

Ovarian cancer begins somewhere beyond the realms of the visible, deep within the body, hidden away out of view of what it is that science can detect. Unless an MRI, CT scan or blood test is done, ovarian cancer goes unnoticed. Ovarian cancer is a great deceiver. Ovarian cancer is almost always a death sentence. Williams' refusal to leave her mother's side as she begins the death process is the unbearable story of witnessing a fading out of life. What traces of life are left toward the end stage of ovarian cancer are difficult to capture in language. The trace, Derrida (1976) states, is the "arche-phenomenon of 'memory'" (p. 70). Williams' mother becomes, in the end, a memory-trace, like the disappearance of birds.

Derrida (1976) remarks that the entire history of Western philosophy has eradicated any notion akin to the trace, because it is steeped in what he calls a metaphysics of presence. Western philosophy cannot handle its Other: the Other of the void, which begins perhaps with a trace. Even though in ancient Greek thought the void was a topic that was discussed among many of the pre-Socratics as well as contemporaries of Plato, later philosophers like Lucretius and Epicurus, the void vanished with the rise of scientism during the Enlightenment. Systematic philosophy—like Euclidean geometry—served to enclose concepts inside of systems—or grids—so as to make things neat and tidy. Concepts like the void or the trace could not be boxed in or systematized. The enigmatic, then, was eliminated from Enlightenment narratives. Derrida (1976) states that the rise of Euclidean-like systems—Enlightenment narratives—reified dualisms. But dualisms—in the history of Western philosophy—can be traced back to Parmenides, an ancient Greek philosopher who carved the world up into dualisms. Plato was enamored of Parmenides; some suggest that Plato's dualistic theory of ideas was borrowed from Parmenides. Plato even devoted an entire dialog to Parmenides. However, dualisms are highly problematic because this world is far more complex than this/or that world. Derrida (1976) remarks:

All dualisms, all theories of the immortality of the soul or of the spirit, as well as all monisms, spiritualist or materialist, dialectical or vulgar, are the unique theme of a metaphysics whose entire history was compelled to strive toward the reduction of the trace. (p. 71)

What philosophers could not contain—i.e. the idea of the trace—they neatly put away in closed systems. Those things which slipped beyond systems, those things which slipped beyond the Euclidian grid, were put under erasure.

It is interesting to note, however, that slippery concepts like the void or the clinamen (meaning the swerve and chance happenings of atoms) formulated by Lucretius and Epicurus, got hidden away in the fold of the history of philosophy until they were resurrected, mostly by French postmodern thinkers such as Michel Serres (2001) Alain Badiou (2009), Althusser (2006), to name but a few. But schools such as The Vienna Circle, namely the analytic tradition of philosophy—which still dominates philosophy continue to put under erasure that which is slippery. Philosophy of science is dominated by subjects like probability theory, mathematical logic and AI. The poetic in philosophy—i.e. the notion of the trace—is not recognized by mainstream philosophers, who seem to want to imitate their scientific colleagues.

Adorno's (1966/2007) "nonconceptualities" (p. 11) make philosophers anxious. Recall, Adorno argued that philosophy should point toward what it is not. Philosophy, in other words, needs to get beyond the conceptual and venture into more obscure realms, or venture into the non-philosophical so as to speak to non-philosophers. Adorno's work on music and politics are good examples of what he means by philosophy getting beyond the conceptual. If philosophy is to have meaning outside the sphere of professional philosophers, it must speak to a broader audience. Still, today this is an ongoing debate and problem for philosophy as a discipline. Walter Benjamin's (2006) notion of the aura, and his more mystical concepts in the *Philosophy of History*, explore concepts that cannot easily be contained or even explained. The aura is a good example of the nonconceptual; the aura is a slippery concept that cannot be signified, explained or contained. Original artworks, Benjamin argued, had an aura about them. For Benjamin, the problem is the loss of aura once artworks become "mechanically reproduced." Of course this point is debatable, but here the point is that the concept of the aura opens philosophy to that which is slippery.

Death—as an experience—that is not a concept. Of course, death is a concept one can think about philosophically. But the occurrence of death is beyond the conceptual. One cannot think of one's own death. Death—as it is experienced—is perhaps one of the most slippery non-concepts (to draw on Adorno), for it is nearly impossible to say what death is. Even in medical terms, physicians do not know—exactly—what death is.

(Male) philosophers have historically been uncomfortable with issues around the body and emotions: what they cannot capture in words. Philosophy is a good place to hide in intellectualism, when emotions are too much to bear. Perhaps this is why many mainstream philosophers have contempt for psychoanalysis. This pandora's box of emotions is almost too much for philosophers who like to live in concepts only, without bodies. More postmodern (French) philosophers, however, have made a move toward Lacanian psychoanalysis in the intersections of philosophy.

Death on the Horizon: Terry Tempest Williams' Unease

Terry Tempest Williams—in writing about the way in which she intuits that her mother is dying—states: "It's strange to feel change coming. It's easy to ignore. An underlying restlessness seems to accompany it like birds flocking before a storm. We go about our business with the usual alacrity, while in the pit of our stomach there is a sense of something tenuous" (p. 24). Williams intuits that her mother is very ill; Williams knows on a gut level, in fact, that her mother is dying. This unease lends to the feeling that, as Adorno (2008) puts it, "all is not well with the world" (p. 20). Adorno (2008) states:

> Can thought bear the idea that a given reality is meaningless and that the mind is unable to orient itself; or whether the intellect has become so enfeebled that it finds itself paralysed [sic] by the idea that all is not well with the world (p. 20)

Williams' intuits early on that something is terribly wrong with her mother. Many people sense a kind of unease when death looms, but denial—as a psychological defense mechanism—becomes reified, so as to keep psyche from collapsing. Denial—a concept of great importance for Freud—is a common response for those experiencing a traumatic event.

In relation to covid—and the poor outcomes of those who are not vaccinated—denial is a common defense mechanism, faced with the possibility of dying. When physicians break the bad news to families, that their loved ones is about to be put on a ventilator, an initial response tends to be this is not happening. I have heard families utter these words over and over, as they face the fact that their loved ones could die from covid. Even at the very end of life, when families see their loved ones on ventilators because of covid (through web ex), they still cannot believe what is happening and tend to go into denial. Denial is a very powerful defense mechanism, but it can also become detrimental in not facing up to the truth. Before covid patents are put on ventilators, some argue with medical professionals that they do not have covid, or that covid is not real.

Turning a bad situation into something that it is not—like saying to a patient all will be well, or your son will be going to a better place, i.e. heaven—or turning things into their opposite (another Freudian form of denial), does not help, but only makes things worse. A death that did not have to happen is, in the end, without meaning, or as Adorno (2008) puts it "meaningless." When medical professionals say that these deaths were unnecessary, meaningless, what they are suggesting is that many covid deaths—for example—did not have to happen. The meaninglessness of these deaths that did not have to happen is what gets misunderstood by many. It is easier to think that God has a grand plan for all, that this was destiny, or that this happened for a reason are all defense mechanisms. When Lucretius and Epicurus wrote about the concept of the clinamen or the swerve—in the realm of atoms—what they were suggesting is that nothing is destined to happen, that all is chance. That the world came to be at all was a chance occurrence—that atoms crashed into each other and from that built a world of life was probably an accident of nature, not caused by a prime mover or God, or destiny or reason. I have found in my clinical work as a chaplain that the majority of patients I have witnessed dying do not believe that chance has much to do with anything. The idea that all is destiny, or that there is a reason for everything, is a common belief. I suppose it is, in a way, easier to think that there is a reason for everything. But dying from covid is a good example of a chance occurrence. It is by chance that one becomes ill from covid. Even if vaccinated, covid can slip through the cracks and make you sick. Take all the precautions you wish but covid will still find a way to invade your body. For some, the chances of getting covid are higher because they are immune-suppressed, even if precautions are taken. Still, chance occurrences play a part in getting covid. All it takes is a few seconds of being in the wrong place at the wrong time and breathing in something that the body cannot tolerate. The virus does not have a reason; it just is.

But, again as a chaplain I have found that more often than not most cannot deal with a thought like this, so they fabulate a meaning—a reason—where there is none. Families often resort to religious cliches, or Liebnizian ideas that God willed this, or that it's all for the best because the patient will no longer suffer, or that God is taking someone "home." Falling back upon religious cliches is so common as to be baffling. But given the strength of defense mechanisms, the belief in these cliches should not be surprising. Cliches gloss over hard truths that people cannot bear.

When Terry Tempest Williams' (2001) mother realizes that she is dying, she states: "I am facing my own mortality—again—something I thought I had already done twelve years ago. Do you know how strange it is to know your days are limited? To have no future" (p. 28)? It is unthinkable—unbearable—to think that one has "no future." For the witness, The Other's death is wholly other to experience, to understanding or comprehension. But facing one's own death differs radically from witnessing the death of the Other. Levianas (2000) cites Epicurus who famously stated, "If you are there, then death is not there; if it is there, you are not there" (p. 19). Death is the most difficult thing to think because one simply cannot think it. One cannot think one's own nothingness. One cannot think the Other's nothingness either. At the moment of death of the Other, the witness still cannot think the nothingness of the Other's death. There is a time—a strange time of denial—at that moment of death. The hardest part of witnessing the Other's death—for many—is leaving the body. To leave the body means, in a way, to accept that the person is no longer there, that the body is just that. I have heard many times family members—after the death of a loved one say—I cannot leave her there. How can I leave her here? This is perhaps the most excruciatingly painful moment in the death experience for those left behind. But covid makes the situation worse because family members are not at the bedside. Family members might be on the phone with the chaplain, or looking through a computer screen while the patient dies. This makes the acceptance of the death all the more difficult because the scene is so surreal.

Witnessing the death of the Other because of covid—through that computer screen—is, indeed, what radical alterity means. No one can understand or comprehend the end of an other's life. But covid magnifies the horrors of death and the inhumane situation families must endure because they cannot be there at the bedside with their loved ones. Often those who are left behind turn to the chaplain for answers. I have had people ask me things like: why did this happen? Those who are left behind often engage in magical thinking and have even turned to me, the chaplain, and have said things like "Can't you bring him back?" It is an astonishing question. The chaplain—some believe—has magical powers, or has some connection with God others do not have. It is simply astonishing—again—to think that many people believe these things, especially at the moment of death when families are feeling so utterly desperate and torn apart. Those who are left behind want answers that I cannot give. How to respond to the death of the Other, the Otherness of that death?

Diat (2019) states: " I would like… to offer some hope, because the monks show us that a humane death is possible. Twenty-first century man is not condemned to lonely endings, without love, in anonymous hospital rooms" (p. 13). Diat (2019), like all of us, could not anticipate that there would come a time in modern history when (covid) deaths are indeed "inhumane" and that they get played out "without love, in anonymous hospital rooms" (p. 13).

The other horrifying thing about covid deaths is that as soon as one covid patient dies and they are wrapped up in plastic, taken to the morgue to be put into refrigerator storage for 48 hours—because they are still contagious after two days, even after death—the next covid patient is wheeled into the same room to face the very same ending. Death on the covid ward has become a kind of Ford-like factory: one body comes in and dies; the next body comes in and dies; the next body comes in and dies. At the height of the pandemic during the first year, I witnessed body-bags being taken in and out of covid rooms as if on a conveyer-belt. For a time there was a lull in the numbers of covid patients and covid deaths on the covid floors. But in 2022 the uptick in covid deaths has increased and the conveyer-belt of death has started up again, body bad after body bag after body bag. Physicians and nurses, respiratory therapists and chaplains report that they have never—in their lifetimes—experienced anything like the covid crisis. And, as a matter of fact the covid crisis has created another crisis: a terrible shortage of healthcare workers. Many nurses have quite the profession altogether: the deaths are just overwhelming. In 2022, the thing that has changed so radically is that now children are ending up in pediatric ICUs and even in neonatal ICUs. The medical staff—who have never seen so many children die—are beyond the breaking point. There is perhaps nothing worse than watching a child suffer and die. Covid is merciless.

In the beginning of the pandemic there was much concern about how to clean covid hallways and rooms. But when the deaths were coming faster than the medical staff could handle, the cleaning of the rooms became rushed, and then minimal. There just wasn't time between patients to clean the rooms as they might have been cleaned during non-covid times. In the beginning of the covid crisis in 2020, yellow tape—not unlike crime scene tape—was draped around the hallways until the hallways could be adequately cleaned. But after a while the yellow tape disappeared because there simply wasn't time to take time between deaths to clean the hallways. I once asked a nurse when the pandemic was all over how they will sanitize the covid wards: his answer was, "I don't know, they probably won't because nobody knows how to sanitize this place against covid."

Facing A Psychic Sibera

Terry Tempest Williams' (2001) mother said to her: "Each of us must face our own Siberia... No one can rescue us. My cancer is my Siberia" (p. 93). There is nothing lonelier than knowing that one is going to die, imminently, from cancer, or covid for that matter. Siberia—a metaphor for a psychic state of total aloneness when nearing death—is not something we like to think about. Williams' mother says also that no one can "rescue" her. A natural response to someone who is dying is the wish to rescue them from their emotional pain. But that is not at all helpful, in reality. The work of the chaplain is to allow the dying patient to feel the pain associated with dying and not offer rescue fantasies or false hope. Rescue fantasies are just that, fantasies. "Can't you bring him back?" The magical thinking that is often shared with chaplains is an example of a rescue fantasy. Somehow, people want to be rescued from that which they cannot face. But death is something that one must face alone, without gloss or rescue.

Joan Didion

Joan Didion's (2005) *Year of Magical Thinking* is an unbearable story of compounded grief. Didion's husband and daughter both died within a short span of time, one after the other. When someone experiences multiple deaths like Didion did, and one attempts to cope or not, with multiple tragedies, this is what is referred to as compounded grief.

I want to focus here, however, on Didion's response to her husband's death. It was his death that began what she called her *year of magical thinking*. A common response immediately after someone dies is that people report that they think that they see the person who has died everywhere; this is a form of magical thinking. Magical thinking is a defense mechanism against the utter collapse of the psyche, especially after the death of a loved one. In Didion's case, she reports that this kind of thinking was prolonged—for an entire year. This might seem like an uncommon form of magical thinking—because of the duration—but it is not uncommon at all. Processing death takes time; the grieving process differs for everyone. Sometimes it does take years to process; sometimes deaths are never processed. Grief can last a lifetime. There are some wounds that never heal. Psychologists might call this pathological, but I think not. That we are supposed to get over the death of a loved one is perhaps magical thinking in and of itself.

The thought that the dead are gone—forever—is just too much to bear. It is nearly impossible to cope with, especially early on after the death happens. The forever-ness of death is impossible to think. Some fundamentalist Christians believe that death is not forever and that upon their own death, they will see others in their family who have died. This belief serves to console and to un-do death because it is too unbearable to think. Of course, no one knows what happens after death, but the probability that other dead relatives are waiting at the gates of heaven is rather unlikely. And this is the problem with belief; it can become a form of magical thinking. Glossing over the truth which is too hard to bear, is, again, a defense mechanism against pain. When I first began my work as a chaplain, I was astonished to learn how many people believe that death is not real; on the other side—they say—the dead will be waiting for them with open arms.

Joan Didion's (2005) memoir begins with four powerful sentences that she repeats throughout her memoir, as if trying to work through her grief. Didion states:

> Life changes fast.
> Life changes in the instant.
> You sit down to dinner and life as you know it ends.
> The question of self-pity. (p. 3)

Derrida (1995) points out that "when one repeats a traumatism, Freud teaches us, one is trying to get control of it" (p. 382). Didion repeats the above mantra throughout her memoir with special attention to the lines: "You sit down to dinner and life as you know it ends" (p. 3). The power of this sentence overwhelms. Didion's figurative speech is more powerful than literally describing what happens to a man having a heart attack while at the dinner table.

Didion's husband died of sudden cardiac arrest; he just seemed to slump over at the dinner table. And then he was dead. Part of what makes this so awful is where he died: at the dinner table. Didion (2005) remarks that "It was in fact the ordinary nature of everything preceding the event that prevented me from truly believing it had happened" (p. 4). As a chaplain, I have heard similar stories many times. I recall a family member saying to me something to the effect that her father was fine one minute and dead the next. How could that have happened? Or, it all started with a tickle in his throat. Then came the cough, the hospitalization, the intubation, the ventilator and death. Covid deaths sometimes happen like this. Sometimes, covid deaths come on quickly and the situation becomes grave quickly. A man walks into the emergency room and he is dead two days later. Covid can kill quickly. Or, sometimes covid deaths linger; they happen over a period of a few weeks, sometimes months.

The covid crisis began with a few patients, maybe four. Then there were ten patients. Then an entire wing of the hospital; then the birth of covid wards, then multiple floors of covid patients; then covid patients spilling out onto the general hospital floors. Shortly after that there were no more ICU rooms and the hospital was at capacity. It all happened slowly and quickly seemingly all at once. That was in 2020. After a few months things calmed down, we were back down to four patients, then two. And then none. And a few months passed and it started all over again but worse. The second year of the pandemic brought with it more severe illness, younger patients, more deaths. Fewer patients went home. The hospital at capacity, no more ICU rooms and the refrigerator trucks tucked away in a hidden recess of the hospital. The morgue was full. It happened in slow motion and yet all at once, as if time itself went crazy. In 2022 things got worse, even still. More covid deaths, younger children died. Healthcare workers began getting sick; some died by suicide. The covid crisis unfolding before our eyes was almost unbelievable. It is not hard to imagine why magical thinking becomes necessary when faced with unprecedented levels of trauma.

Levinas (2000) writes about the "duration of time" (p. 7)—a notion that he perhaps borrows from Henri Bergson's (2015) notion of *duree*, which means duration in relation to time. Bergson (2015) points out the difference between what he calls "homogeneous time" (p. 90) against what he calls "heterogeneity which is the very ground of our experience" (p. 97). It does seem on one level that time is felt as a duration, a smooth flowing "homogeneous" experience, as moments flow one into the next. But that is not really how time works. The sensation of time passing is so complex and to get into what time is in any depth goes beyond the scope of this book. However, one might say that the experience of time can be felt in both "homogeneous" and "heterogeneous" ways simultaneously. Or, time can feel as if it has stopped altogether.

When something traumatic happens, like Didion's husband dying from a sudden cardiac arrest at the dinner table, it would seem that time just stopped altogether. In a world of magical thinking the experience of time changes. Magical thinking suggests the ability to go backwards in time, in order to bring someone back from the dead. If I just imagine my father enough, maybe he will come back; I can imagine him back to life. This is not an uncommon feeling among those who have lost loved ones.

Time moves slowly when one is ill; time moves quickly when one is deeply engaged in a project. Simultaneity of time(s) is felt when one thinks of something in the past—the death of a loved one, say—while in the present. The past sometimes can overwhelm the present. This, Freud called melancholy. Getting stuck in the past because of melancholy is like turning into a rock, Freud suggested. Moving beyond melancholy—beyond petrification—through what Freud called *the work of mourning* gets one unstuck in time and memory. But when in the middle of a terrible situation, like Joan Didion's unbearable story of losing both her husband and daughter in a very short amount of time, mourning work becomes impossible. If one cannot get beyond melancholy and grief, Didion (2005) points out that psychologists refer to this as "pathological bereavement" (p. 48). But what makes bereavement pathological? To say that there is a certain amount of time one has in order to get over the dead is a ridiculous idea. But it is widely believed that if you can't get over your grief, there is something wrong with you. Right after 9/11, news anchors resorted to the easy cliches of moving on, getting over this, and getting back to normal. I recall how astounded I was just how quickly news anchors resorted to this kind of talk. It all seemed ludicrous to me, so American to not handle grief at all and just get over it and move on. American and Disneyfied attitudes about death make grief even worse, especially for those suffering from the loss of mass casualties like 9/11. In the face of a global pandemic, now going into its third year and beyond, Americans want to get back to normal; we are living in an entire culture that has succumbed to magical thinking. Medical experts warn that becoming complacent, pretending that all is well, will result in more deaths. And herein lies the danger of magical thinking. One can, alternatively, use magical thinking as a defense mechanism to keep the psyche intact—for a while—but ongoing use of magical thinking can put life into an arrest, psychically.

Didion (2005) repeats: "Life changes in the instant" (p. 3). Indeed, it does. Covid seems to have come out of nowhere. In the beginning of the pandemic, they said, it will not come here. Well, it did. "Life changes in an instant." It seemed that all of a sudden everybody was dying. Didion states: *"You sit down to dinner and life as you know it ends.* [italics in the original]. *In a heartbeat"* (p. 63). You wake up with a pain in your abdomen one day only to learn that you have ovarian cancer. Life changes, yes, in a heartbeat. I have spent my entire adult life studying philosophy. They say that death is the philosopher's stone. Philosophy prepares one for death, they say. But that too is magical thinking. One day I woke up with pain in my abdomen only to find out that I had ovarian cancer. In a moment my life changed. I know my days are numbered, as are everyone's. But living with ovarian cancer is akin to living with a gun to one's head, as Flannery O'Conner might put it. I tell the chief medical officer of the hospital that the reason I became a chaplain is because one day I woke up and my life changed in an instant. It was a freezing cold February in 2016. I woke up with a pain in my abdomen. My life changed forever. I became a chaplain after surviving, but who knows for how long. Nobody knows when death will call.

Maurice Merleau-Ponty (2010) states: "I nevertheless live in an atmosphere of death in general, and there is a kind of essence of death always on the horizon of my thinking. In short, just as the instant of my death is a future to which I have no access, so I am necessarily destined never to live through the presence of another to himself" (p. 424). Didion cannot, as Merleau-Ponty points out, "live through the presence" of her husband's death. No one can die your death for you. "At the instant" of death nobody knows what happens. The "instant of death" is unthinkable. The witness cannot understand the instant of death either. When the Other dies, those agonizing moments of deathly silence fill the air. That instant of death is beyond signification.

Joan Didion attempts to understand her husband's experience in that instant to no avail. Didion (2005) reports the facts of her husband's death—as if it were a police report—. She states the facts: here is what happened but I still do not understand what happened. I should understand because here is what happened, here are the facts. Didion (2005) remarks:

> Nine months and five days ago, at approximately nine o'clock in the evening of December 30, 2003, my husband John Gregory Dunne, appeared to (or did) experience, at the table where he and I just sat down to dinner in the living room of our apartment in New York, a sudden massive coronary event that caused his death. (p. 7)

Didion writes about her husband's death stating the facts of the case. Stating the facts of the case—as detailed as they may be—still do not help Didion understands what has occurred. The instant of a death cannot be understood by a verbatim description that led up to that instant. Didion juxtaposes police-like statements above with magical thinking later on when she declares: "I needed to be alone so that he could come back" (p. 33).

Magical thinking—like Didion's—is a kind of differance, as Derrida (1976) would put it; magical thinking "defers—differs" (p. 66). Magical thinking, that is, delays understanding and defers meaning. Something that one cannot currently process or understand—like death—delays understanding, delays meaning, and holds meanings at bay. That perhaps later one will understand or that one will never understand a death, is what differance means. Derrida's notion of differance might seem abstract but it actually is not. To delay understanding or to delay meaning does not necessarily mean that one day understanding will arrive. Sometimes—especially around death—understanding never arrives. Derrida's (1976) notion of differance is not easy to understand in and of itself; nor is it easy to explain. One can see, though, how useful the concept of differance is when thinking about death and all especially in the context of magical thinking. Engaging in magical thinking mixes up time and space, imagination and reality.

Ironically, Didion's (2005) disbelief and anguish only worsen when she is in the company of a priest. She states:

> *But I did the ritual. I did it all.* I did St. John the Divine, I did the chant in Latin, I did the Catholic priest and the Episcopal priest.... *And it still didn't bring him back.* [all italics in the original]. (p. 43)

A primary emotion for those who experience the death of the Other is rage: chaplains often get the brunt of the rage because we are right there. Rage has to go somewhere and it is often directed at the chaplain or priest. Why can't you bring him back? But I thought? I have witnessed family members becoming so angry, in fact, after a loved one dies that they throw chairs, attempt to punch the chaplains, spit at the chaplains, curse and scream at the top of their lungs and so on. Rage is part of the grief process and is to be expected. But rage against the priest and or chaplain is quite shocking. And this is part of the problem of magical thinking: that priests and chaplains have magical powers to resurrect the dead.

In cases of covid when families experience multiple deaths from this disease, rage and violence come later; it is delayed and can become quite dangerous. In fact, there has been a radical uptick in gun violence and killings since covid began. Of course, murder is much more complicated than saying it has one cause, like covid. Part of the reason why so many have resorted to gun violence in the United States has to do with the inability to manage emotions, especially when a loved one dies. Where there are guns, there will be violence, and sometimes murders. The pandemic rages on in invisible violence as the virus steals lives day in and day out seemingly without end. No amount of magical thinking can stop covid.

Derrick Jensen

Jensen's (2000) unbearable story differs from Terry Tempest Williams' (2001) story and Joan Didion's (2005) story in that it is not about death and dying but it is about the killing of a spirit. There are many ways to kill someone's spirit. Paul Schreber in *My Nervous Illness* had a phrase that was later taken up by Deleuze and Guattari (2000) in *Anti-Oedipus*, and that phrase was "soul murder." Jensen's unbearable story is a multilayered trauma as he and his brother, sister and mother were beaten and raped by his father. But Jensen says that the physical abuse was not the worst of it. Jensen reports what was worse was his father's gaslighting. Jensen's father simply pretended that nothing happened. No rapes occurred, and no one was beaten. Jensen's father attempted to undo reality.

Jensen's abusive father—like so many abusive parents—resorts to gaslighting, a technique to make others feel like their reality isn't real and that what has happened—the acts of abuse—never happened. Gaslighting is a way to erase reality. That erasure—in and of itself—Jensen remarks, is the worst part of abuse. The undoing of reality, continued and sustained lies, made Jensen's entire life a search for the truth. Jensen reports that his emotions were numbed due to all the abuse he endured as a child; he fights as an adult to get back his feelings that he numbed as a child; to re-find his home in himself and in nature. Like Terry Tempest Williams, Jensen takes refuge in nature. And like Terry Tempest Williams, Jensen is an ecological activist. Jensen—like Williams—became a writer and social activist, an ecologist and public intellectual. Jensen (2000) argues in his book that the abuse he endured as a child is reflective of a larger culture of abuse—in the United States—that is perpetuated by those in power, by what Adorno (1966/2007) called the "administered world" (p. 20). The administered world is a Kafkaesque nightmare, where petty bureaucrats ruin the world. Petty bureaucrats who hold power and wield power over against those they fear—is something about which Kafka wrote.

Although Jensen's father was an attorney, and not a petty bureaucrat, he was still an administrator of the law, an officer of the court, and misused his power to kill the spirit of his entire family. Jensen, again, makes a connection between ecological devastation and the devastation of the family. Devastation of lives begins at home. Global warming and the pandemic go hand in glove, some argue. Ecological activists argue that it is no accident that the collision of covid and our current ecological crisis have arrived seemingly all at once.

Jensen's father brutalized his family—through raping and beating, humiliating and pretending that none of that occurred. Jensen (2000) states that "we learned, day after day, that we could not trust our perceptions, and that we were better off not listening to our emotions. Daily we forgot, and if a memory pushed its way to the surface we forgot again" (p. 3).

Early on in this book, I discussed issues of perception and what I called puzzles of perception. I drew upon Ludwig Wittgenstein's (1958) example of the duck-rabbit, a drawing by one Jastrow. The duck-rabbit puzzle—recall—is one of perception: if one looks at the duck-rabbit one way, a rabbit emerges. If one looks again at the duck-rabbit another way, a duck emerges. Duck or rabbit? It depends on how you look at it. What is most curious, though, is that it is impossible to see both the duck and the rabbit at the same time. Perceptions are tricky and complicated.

Now, imagine that one's perception is so undone by so much violence that upon looking at the picture of the duck-rabbit, neither the duck nor the rabbit emerges at all. The victim of abuse might see, rather, a tangle of lines that are meaningless. When one's perceptions are so thoroughly obliterated through violence—in the case of Jensen—what seems to others like a child's play to some, like the duck-rabbit game—becomes an utter impossibility to others. The duck-rabbit then is no longer a game or puzzle of perception because perception is utterly obliterated. Thus, the larger question here is how does one move through the world with an obliterated sense of perception of anything at all? What might seem easy for others to perceive becomes impossible for those whose perceptions are no longer intact.

Another analogy of this would be blindness. If one woke up one day and could not see anything, the loss of sight also means a loss of perception through vision. This is an extreme example but it might help to clarify what it is I am attempting to say here. Or, take the case of sudden color blindness. One day a world of colors opens out onto the horizon; the next day the world has turned completely grey. Or take the case of the inability to recognize faces of familiar people, or musicians who suddenly lose the ability to read music. Oliver Sacks (2010) has written extensively about many different kinds of perceptual problems in his book *The Mind's Eye* in his work as a neurologist.

Violence can also alter perceptions in a way that makes the world, quite simply, unrecognizable. The earlier violence is done, the harder it is to repair. The inability to perceive things is not only neurological; it is also emotional, as Freud well knew. The inability to trust one's perceptions at all—as Jensen (2000) points out—creates life-long problems in terms of building trust.

Freud argued throughout his work that when one grows up in an abusive household—whether the abuse is physical or emotional, or both— unconsciously—the psyche seeks out the same kinds of experiences in other relationships later in life. The psyche does what is familiar; it seeks the familiar, even if that familiar is harmful. This is called negative transference or what Freud called the death drive. There is a self-destructive element at work in relationships—unconsciously driven—especially if destructive relations are familiar. The unconscious seeks out the violence that one experienced as a child. This is also referred to as repetition compulsion by Freud.

Jensen (2000) states that the worst of his father's abuse came not in the physical violence but in his absolute "denial that any of it even occurred" (p. 3). This denial is what makes people feel crazy because they can no longer trust their sense of reality at all. Did that not happen? That is the question Jensen raises throughout his book. How could that have happened? If Jensen's father continually denied that the violence and repeatedly lied about what he had done, after a while the lies seem as if they are true. This creates a confusing world for a child.

Former President Trump is the master of gaslighting; not only did he gaslight his family, he gaslighted an entire nation. The term gaslighting has now become a common word in our everyday conversations. Before Trump's presidency, this word was used mostly by psychologists to deal with situations of child abuse and the experiences that Jensen describes.

Hannah Arendt (1994) wrote extensively about cultural gaslighting—without using the term—as she described how the Nazis gaslit, not only a nation, but mostly all of Europe. It is important to note that it wasn't only Germany that went along with Hitler's genocidal program; there were at least twelve or more collaborating countries that aided Hitler and conspired against the Jewish people. Arendt (1994) explains that the way in which Hitler operated went even beyond typical fascist techniques. Arendt (1994) states:

> The essential characteristic of fascist propaganda was never its lies, for this is something more or less common to propaganda everywhere and of every time. The essential thing was that they [the Nazis] exploited the age-old Occidental prejudice which confuses reality with truth, and made that "true" which until then could only be stated as a lie. It is for this reason that any argumentation with fascists—the so-called counter-propaganda—Is so extremely senseless.... (pp. 146-147)

Arendt's claim that arguing with fascists is senseless rings true today with Trump loyalists: they just do not want to believe in the truth; the live lies. Trump loyalists, still after three years of covid, do not believe it is real; they are what has become known as anti-vaxxers, up until the day they die—of covid, still believing that covid does not exist. Trying to argue with an anti-vaxxer is, as Arendt said of fascists—"extremely senseless" because they simply do not listen to the truth.

Again, to reiterate, Jensen's (2000) overarching thesis of his book is not merely about his family and the violence he endured growing up; he states emphatically that the family is a mirror of the larger (abusive) culture. What happens in families happens in cultures. And perhaps the culture of a country, in turn, influences what happens in families. Families are cultural phenomena; families are built upon and socially constructed out of the larger culture into which they are thrown, if you will. What Jensen's father perpetuated upon his family was always already a part of Western culture.

Of course American history is very different from that of Europe, but still we have inherited many European traditions, and certainly our schooling system is based on the Prussian system. It is a well-known fact that Prussian schools were noted for their sadistic pedagogues. Sadistic pedagogues are probably sadistic parents as well. Although the United States has a unique culture and history, that culture and history did not come from nowhere.

The cultural violence both Jensen and Arendt write about can also be applied to our current American political situation, even after Trump has left office. As I remarked earlier, the gaslighting continues and Arendt's description of the way in which truth is turned into lies is applicable to what many in the American government—especially in the United States Senate—are doing especially about the January 6, 2021 insurrection. It is remarkable that so many Republican senators say things like the insurrection did not happen, that what we saw on television on that fateful day was little more than a tourist visit. This whitewashing of history, history put under erasure, is beyond Orwellian. And these lies persist into 2022; Trump is still spinning lies about the "stolen" election and people still—remarkably—believe him. Sinclair Lewis wrote a book in the 1930s titled *It Can't Happen Here*. He knew, indeed, that it can happen here and will happen here. That is, fascism was always-already here in the 1930s. It was just a matter of time before pandora's box was opened. The problem is, how do we shut that box? Can we shut Trump out of the picture—ever—or his minions? Or will the Trump era live-on? Isn't it time we cut Trump out of public life?

Jensen (2000) tells us that he finally decided to completely cut his father out of his life forever. This is a remarkably brave move. Most children stand by their parents, even if they were brutally beaten and abused; children—even if they were abused—sometimes protect their parents from prosecution. Secrecy is a problem in families of abuse. But Jensen never wanted to cover over his father's crimes or protect him in any way; Jensen does not keep family secrets from the public: Jensen holds nothing back.

Jensen (2000) asks: "refined in a crucible of violence, how can you ever think of carrying on" (p. 240)? Jensen's entire life project is—to carry on—despite the violence he endured as a child. His life project is to tell the truth about what happened. What makes Jensen's work so important is that he makes the connection between family violence and cultural violence. The ecosphere is the larger cultural site of destruction and violence: the destruction that happens inside of families spills out into the ecosphere. Capitalist greed and callous attitudes toward the earth and her creatures go hand in glove with violence on the micro and macro levels of family and culture. Global warming is a direct result of this violence and it will be the end of all of us; ecologists know that extinction is not far off if we do not change what we are doing. These are the "inconvenient truths" that Al Gore (2006) wrote about some time ago. And yes, they are "inconvenient" especially for developers who are only interested in making profits and lining their own pockets at the expense of the health of the planet and her creatures. These "inconvenient truths" are now coming home to bear as fires in the West are burning in ways we have never seen before, as temperatures are rising so high that some countries are creating manufactured rain to cool things down, that hurricanes and tornadoes, tsunamis and earthquakes are getting worse, year by year. The global pandemic—Jensen would say—goes hand in glove with ecological devastation. Not that pandemics are new, they are not. Adorno stated that "The splinter in your eye" (cited in Jay) which, as Martin Jay (2020) reminds, is "the best magnifying glass" because.... "it cannot be ignored" (p. xii). The pandemic is the "splinter in the eye" that cannot be ignored.

Jensen's (2000) splinter in his eye is his father and what violence his father did to his family. Jensen (2000), in a shocking passage, tells us of one event that especially stands out in his memory:

> My brother's epilepsy, from blows to the head, is among the least of his problems. Having been struck so hard that your brain is damaged in that way, how can you ever create a life? (p. 240)

As a chaplain I have seen children arrive in the emergency room as young as five months old who have brain damage due to being thrown against the wall by a parent. Most parents who bring their children to the emergency room who do things like this—and there are many as shocking as that is—tell the attending physicians tall tales like, my son fell over the couch and hit his head on the floor. The coroner discovers the truth through the autopsy; the guilty parent is then arrested. It is quite shocking that parents do such violence to their children. Jensen's (2002) unbearable story is all too familiar to those who work in pediatric ICUs. Most of the children who are brought in are victims of family violence. And the pandemic has made family violence worse. The pandemic has made things are so hopeless that many resort to violence.

Two brothers owned a barber shop. The pandemic hit, they lost all of their customers, and they lost their business. One of the brothers shot himself in the head and died. I was there as the chaplain to pick up the pieces, but there was nothing I could do or say. This tragedy stands out in my memory because this happened early on when the pandemic first began. Why suicide? Brothers. One survived. The other did not. Why? What could I say?

Jensen (2000) states: "I have grown to understand that in the shadow of the unspeakable I can and must speak" (p. 61). Unbearable stories must be told. Silence is not the answer. Thomas Merton (1966) speaks to the unspeakable as he states:

> The Unspeakable. What is this? Surely, an eschatological image. It is the void that we encounter.... It is the void that contradicts everything that is spoken even before the words are said. (p. 4)

It is better to let the unspeakable speak rather than offer meaningless consolations. It is better to say nothing than reply in easy cliches.

6

The Unbearable Stories of Anton Boisen, Louise DeSalvo and John Gunther

Anton Boisen (1952) wrote his memoir *The Experience of the Inner World: A Study of Mental Disorder and Religious Experience* to describe being hospitalized for a seeming mental collapse. This book is not well known among curriculum scholars, if it is known at all. I highlight Boisen's work in an attempt to bring him back into the archive. Boisen's (1952) work might be unknown to many but I think his work is on par with William James (1958); it is in a similar genre as James' *The Varieties of Religious Experience*. Both men explore their own psychic explorations with breakdown and renewal through religious experience. Here, I will focus on Boisen (1952) and make some remarks about James in relation to Boisen's work.

Boisen is most well-known for his founding of hospital chaplaincy. He came to found this discipline through his own experience as a hospitalized psychiatric patient dealing with a mental crisis and subsequent religious breakthrough. Boisen was hospitalized in the 1920s because he had what seemed to be a psychotic break, but he was still lucid enough to record his experiences and write his memoir. Some would interpret Boisen's work as psychological in nature, as he deals with losing touch with reality; others might interpret Boisen's work as religious. Although both the psychological and religious aspects of the book are important to understand, I would like to do a different kind of reading of his text. Although the psychological and religious are crucial to understand Boisen's contributions to hospital chaplaincy, I also think his work has political ramifications. Most, however, do not read his book in this way. Students of chaplaincy, for example, read Boisen's book as a kind of primer and historical document for how and why hospital chaplaincy began in the United States. Of course, Boisen's work is foundational for work in hospital chaplaincy. But as I read his text—from a curriculum perspective—the most crucial aspect of Boisen's work deals with political ramifications in the context of medicine. This interpretation of Boisen's text, however, has nothing to do with bioethics, or science per se. This is an interdisciplinary reading of Boisen for a broad audience who is perhaps not familiar with Boisen or with hospital chaplaincy.

Hospital chaplaincy is what I would consider a curricular world outside of the institution of schooling, or higher education. *Currere*, as defined as lived experience, inside or outside of the schoolhouse, is applicable to what goes on in hospitals between chaplains, patients and medical personnel. Hospital chaplaincy is a relatively unknown world to most curriculum scholars, with the exception perhaps of those whose work dovetails religious studies, theology or pastoral care. Like any curricular world—a place where one becomes educated, either inside or outside of formal institutions—the hospital is inherently political. Hospital chaplaincy is no stranger to politics.

Hospital chaplaincy emerged primarily because Boisen felt that physicians did not listen to him when he was a psychiatric patient. Boisen (1952) remarks that

> Of course I spent much time puzzling about my own case. I tried to get a chance to talk with the doctor about it. In this I met with little success. That particular hospital took the organicist point of view. The doctors did not believe in talking with patients about their symptoms, which they assumed to be rooted in some as yet undiscovered organic difficulty. The longest time I ever got was fifteen minutes.... It was clear that he had neither understanding nor interest in the religious aspect of my problem. (p. 5)

Boisen comments that the key issue at stake was that his doctor thought that his mental collapse was due to an "organic difficulty" (p. 5). Now, that can be interpreted in various ways. It is here that I think that William James' (1958) work on psychiatric and religious issues becomes most helpful in understanding Boisen's situation. James, like Boisen, points out similar problems in medicine. James (1958) refers to what he calls "medical materialism" (p. 29), which could be similar to "organic[ism]" (Boisen, 1952, p. 5). James (1958) felt that when the brain is reduced to the physical, i.e., the material, physicians cannot explore the things about the brain that they do not understand. There is much about the brain that is still not understood. James (1958) called "medical materialism" "simple-minded" (p. 29). When the brain is reduced to the physical, psychological problems are treated physically, either with shock therapy or with medicines.

Freud's talk therapy is of little interest to modern-day psychiatrists as they are no longer trained in the Freudian tradition. With the birth of psychopharmaceuticals, psychiatry moved away from Freud, even though psychiatry was never very long a bedfellow of Freud's to begin with. At any rate, talk therapy is left to psychologists and social workers.

Child psychiatrist and psychoanalyst D. W. Winnicott once commented on the barbarism of shock therapy and suggested that if the brain is reduced to the physical, the only way to treat it is through the physical. Shock therapy is a direct fallout of materialist thinking. Winnicott was horrified by shock therapy and the prevalence of its use. Shockingly, shock therapy is still used today to treat mental illness. Certainly, there is more to the brain than its organic or material essence. Of course, the brain is made of the same substance as the rest of the body; it is organic and material. However, there is more to the story than the material: there is an Otherness to the brain, called psyche. The root of psychology—psyche—means soul. However, academic psychology dropped the soul out of psychology altogether, dropped the psyche out of psychology. And this is the pity of it all: this was Freud's biggest fear about psychoanalysis coming to the shores of America. He knew it would be ruined or destroyed by the materialist bent of American culture.

The mysterious aspects of the mind or psyche, of consciousness and the unconscious, are left out of psychiatric treatment, especially if a patient is hospitalized. The mysterious aspects of the mind and psyche are left to the hospital chaplains and hospital psychologists who take care of patients after they are stabilized. For the most part, hospitals treat psychiatric patients with pharmaceuticals in locked wards. Some psychiatric patients claim that they are treated like criminals: they lose their freedom, they are locked up and some of the patients I have spoken with in my capacity as chaplain know this and resent it. American culture does, indeed, tend to criminalize psychiatric problems. Many people who end up incarcerated do not belong in prison: this is the plight of the mentally ill in the United States.

When patients present with psychological issues such as delusions, hallucinations, psychoses and/ or severe depression, physicians usually resort first to psychotropic drugs and sometimes shock therapy. Care of the psyche, care of the soul, is something that physicians leave to others. Care of the soul is left to the chaplains. But in Boisen's day, hospital chaplaincy did not exist. None of the medical professionals in hospitals—in the 1920s—were trained to care for the psyche, or the soul.

Bosien (1952), after he was hospitalized and released, studied at Andover Theological Seminary as well as Harvard Graduate School and began his journey in founding hospital chaplaincy. Because his doctors did not listen to him or even attempt to understand him, he felt that hospitals needed trained chaplains to listen to patients, whether they got admitted as psychiatric patients or as patients in the general hospital population.

Being ignored by doctors has political ramifications for the medical community. Boisen's (1952) book is, at root, a political commentary on the lack of (emotional and spiritual) care in the medical community. Michel Foucault (1988) remarks that the "dissociation of doctor and patient" (p. 184) is in direct relation to the way in which the irrational—what gets termed mental illness today—got split off during the rise of the Enlightenment. Foucault (1988) argues that what was once called madness—or what is now called mental illness—during the Middle Ages—"was shown… at a distance, under the eyes of a reason that no longer felt any relation to it" (p. 70). Boisen's experience with his doctor—who did not listen to him—has a context and a history. The irrational was of no concern to the medical world, because the irrational has no basis in the physical or the material. Medicine is a discipline based on science, reason, the material. Of course, these things are crucial in diagnosing and curing disease. But there is more to disease than the material. And this is what Freud understood so well. Freud began as a neurologist but became disillusioned with the material basis of that discipline. He knew that there was more to psyche than the material. He was fascinated with hypnosis and the power of suggestion but felt that there was no way to generalize his findings. From hypnosis he developed psychoanalysis because it was a more systematic way of thinking about psychic problems. Boisen's work is based on Freudian psychoanalysis. Today, students (who follow Boisen's methods) in what is called clinical pastoral education are grounded in psychodynamic psychotherapy, an offshoot of classical Freudian analysis.

Hannah Arendt (1978), in the context of discussing the notion of speculation, i.e. reason, and its uses in philosophy, suggests that philosophers have traditionally used speculation—that is the power of reason—to organize and structure a world that is otherwise too unwieldy. In writing about Hegel, for example, Arendt (1978)—who otherwise feels that Hegel's contributions are invaluable—states that when he speculates about the mind and the structures of the mind, his "architectonic organization" (p. 90) becomes problematic in the sense that "speculative reason" and the truth "is real only as a system" (p. 90).

What systematic philosophers do is build worlds that—perhaps unwittingly—erase that which makes for anxiety, or unease. Hegel's systematic treatment of the mind is Euclidian in nature. Hegel—through enormous complexities, antinomies, contradictions, and his famous dialectic method—constructs perhaps one of the most complicated philosophical systems of the mind in the history of philosophy. The problem is that, at the end of the day, Hegel has an answer to the mystery of the mind. Through the strange dialectical movements of thesis, antithesis and synthesis, philosophy of history comes to a final close when it realizes itself in Spirit. Spirit is not personal but impersonal; for Hegel Spirit is a force? Or some kind of mystical something or other that runs throughout history and sweeps people up in its own realization of itself. Hegel's systematic treatment of Spirit is based on reason, logic and will. Spirit moves through those who come to understand Spirit coming to itself through them; self-consciousness is the consciousness of Spirit at work through human history. Avital Ronell (2002) claims that Hegel's conclusion is rather odd; in fact, in a rather harsh critique, she claims that Hegel's conclusion is little more than "stupidity."

Hannah Arendt (1978) pointed out that for Hegel "the mind is at war with itself" (p. 90). Hegel stated this because he thought that any bit of unreason that slips into thought brings danger. The mind needs to be free of unreason but it must fight in a dialectical fashion, through a series of contradictions and unities to get reason free of unreason, to become self-conscious of Spirit, as Spirit comes to know itself as the absolute Idea. It is interesting to note that at some point in Hegel's life he felt as if he were going crazy. Perhaps his philosophical explorations helped him to hide—psychically—in intellectualism. Arendt (1978) interestingly compares Hegel to Heidegger's (1930) work in *Being and Time* where the upshot of his extremely complicated treatise on being and becoming is that Being eclipses beings. This is similar to Hegel's Spirit eclipsing individual minds. Being is becoming for Heidegger—which means that Being is time. So, too, for Hegel, philosophy of history is movement, Spirit, becoming and time.

Speculative fabulation is at work in both Hegel and Heidegger. The problem, however, is most notable in Heidegger because interpreters feel that what Heidegger was really getting at was that Being is some kind of force whose purpose is to eclipse beings (meaning Jewish people). Being is the Germanic force, in other words, that is moving through history in order to eclipse those who do not adhere to the German, Aryan order. Heidegger's legacy is forever tarnished today because of his posthumously published *Black Notebooks* (2017a; 2017b; 2017c). The discovery of these notebooks changed the way in which *Being and Time* has been interpreted and understood. There is no more question as to Heidegger's anti-Semitism; the *Black Notebooks* have clarified what Being and Time really meant: the obliteration of the Jewish people. Of course, one can read *Being and Time* without reading into it these political implications. It can be read purely on an abstract level. But the political fallout from Heidegger's *Black Notebooks*, makes this task all the more difficult.

Hegel, unlike Heidegger, had a different meaning in mind with his philosophy of history, however. Hegel's (1977) *Phenomenology of Spirit* is little more than Christian ideology hiding in philosophic clothes. But more to the point, when speculative fabulations such as Hegel's and Heidegger's occlude the human dimension of life, when reason becomes a kind of circular and systematic Euclidean framework, armor-proof concepts that near mathematical precision, become meaningless in real human life. This is why Kierkegaard took Hegel to task. There is nothing human about Hegel's phenomenology. For Hegel, reason matters; anything outside of reason does not. Spirit matters; anything but Spirit (as a code word for Christianity) matters little and should be kept out of the philosophical lexicon altogether. Hegel and Heidegger—although both contributed greatly to the history of philosophy in their own ways—are highly problematic in light of real-world events, lacking in humanness. This, too, was Marx's complaint about Hegel. But Marx's work draws heavily on Hegel and turns Hegel upside down. It is not the Spirit that is alienated from itself; it is human beings who are alienated from themselves because they are alienated from their labor.

This is a long digression on how speculative fabulation can go astray. But it relates—in general—to the real-world political implications of a doctor's relationship—or not—with a patient. Given that medicine—as a discipline—is a product of Eurocentric, Enlightenment thought—especially as it glorifies reason at the expense of what cannot be explained through reason (like religious or psychic problems)—one can better understand why a doctor would feel justified ignoring a patient's emotional problems. The doctor is the person of reason; the patient, especially one who is having psychic or emotional difficulties—is a person of unreason. Reason and unreason cannot be squared, and thus the doctor ignores the patient because he feels that he cannot communicate with the patient. Hence, the birth of the chaplain through the work of Anton Boisen.

In the case of Boisen— dismissing and ignoring his emotional distress—led to the birth of hospital chaplaincy. Physicians—a profession based on the physical, the physiological—are caught between the "life of the mind"—to draw on Hannah Arendt's (1978) title of her book—and the life of emotions. But physicians are not trained to deal with emotions. Chaplaincy—with its rigorous training, both in the clinical setting and theoretical grounding in psychodynamic psychotherapy, as well as in pastoral care and theology, fills an enormous void in hospital work. This has become especially marked today with the onset of the covid catastrophe. Never before have hospital chaplains been so needed. And yet, the irony is that many hospitals let chaplains go during the pandemic when they need them most because of the financial burdens of taking care of covid patients. This has created a real problem for hospital staff—as they are suffering under enormous duress—as well as for families who have to deal with the end of life situations that are so difficult and so seemingly inhumane as covid wards are isolation wards.

Judith Butler (2019) points out that for Adorno "there is no morality without an "I" (p. 7). The "I" who is addressed-—Butler says—is always already in relation to the Other. Butler (2019) states, "When the "I" seeks to give account of itself, it can start with itself, but it will find that this self is already implicated in a social temporality that exceeds its own capacities for narration" (pp. 7-8). Yes, the self is always in relation to another; the patient is always in relation to someone, and in the case of the hospital, the patient is always in relation to the doctor. But the doctor can only do so much, and is a physician by training, not a priest or a chaplain—someone who is trained to deal with emotions and spirituality. The doctor has some responsibility to treat his patients as human beings, as subjects, and not as objects, or merely diseases. The relationship between the patient and the doctor is also a two-way street. The doctor is always already in relation to his patients. If patients feel diminished because they feel that they are unheard or ignored by their doctor, what then does the doctor become to the patient? An object? An object of ire perhaps. Out of this ire, Boisen creates hospital chaplaincy.

Boisen felt strongly that mental problems are not medical ones, but problems of the spirit or the soul. To medicalize psychic ills is where things went wrong, Boisen argued.

> Wherever this involves severe conflict pathological features are likely also to appear. In some cases the charge of pathology as applied to religious experience is due simply to the failure to recognize that such phenomena as hallucinations spring from the tapping of the deeper levels of the mental life, and they are not necessarily symptomatic of mental disorder but may be creative and constructive. (1952, p. 82)

Boisen claims that what he experienced when he lost touch with reality was not, in fact, mental illness, or a medical problem. Rather, hallucinations result from a spiritual crisis. William James (1958) came to similar conclusions as did Boisen. James (1958) remarks that "our transmarginal consciousness carries us if we follow it to its remoter side" (p. 387). A "transmarginal consciousness" cannot be measured in numbers, or with CT scans. James (1958) states that "medical materialism finishes up Saint Paul by calling his vision on the road to Damascus a discharging lesion of the occipital cortex.... It snuffs out Saint Teresa as an hysteric, Saint Francis of Assisi as a hereditary degenerate. George Fox's spiritual insights were, in reality, little more than "a symptom of a disordered colon" (p. 29). James, indeed, drives home that emotional distress cannot be reduced to bodily malfunctions, to materiality.

The physician and the priest—during the Middle Ages—were compared; both were considered healers. The physician heals the body; the priest heals the soul. It is interesting to note that these two figures—the physician and the priest were thought of as complimentary, not oppositional. But with the rise of scientism, the wedge between science and religion grew more entrenched. This resulted in a schism between the physician and priest. This schism is the root of contempt by the physician for the priest or by the priest for the physician. This contempt, say, on the part of the physician, then is projected onto the patient—perhaps unconsciously—who becomes the object of the physician's visceral no-reaction—to patients who suffer from psychic or spiritual breakdown. When the object of disease cannot be categorized or easily put on a checklist, the physician—again perhaps unconsciously—cannot treat what he is not trained to treat. Ignoring patients' emotional and spiritual crises is, indeed, an act of violence. Butler (2019) suggests that "Adorno helps us to understand that its violence [i.e. the focus on the universal] consists in part in its indifference to the social conditions under which a living appropriation might become possible" (p. 7). I would add that indifference to social conditions which create the very psychic breakdowns patients suffer in the first place—in the context of medicine—is also crucial in understanding a doctor's (non)relation with a patient suffering from a psychic or spiritual collapse.

The reasons for the contempt on both sides of the relationship between physician and priest are highly complex. It is important to note, following Foucault, that relationships between such figures change over time and indeed historicity is important to understand in order to see how these relationships have shifted over centuries. Before the advent of the Enlightenment, theology was considered the crowning discipline. With the rise of the Enlightenment, with Descartes' cogito, with Kant's pure reason, with Hegel's Spirit, with the rise of medicine, theology and the priests lost power and prestige. Today, theology—as well as philosophy—struggles to stay alive within the academy as the humanities as a whole are in trouble. The professional disciplines such as medicine, public health, business, information technology, nursing, education and academic psychology have become more important to universities than the humanities. The Humanities—of which theology is a part—are seen as useless disciplines, mere fluff to fill the time. Business schools bring in capital; philosophy and theology bring in ideas. In the corporate university, ideas seem to matter little. Academic fields tied to the economy—like business—are now the crowning disciplines—in the neo-liberal university, where capital is all and ideas matter little.

Boisen's (1952) dream of hospital chaplaincy—which he began in the late 1920s—is feeling the same trouble as other humanities disciplines in the academy. Hospital chaplaincy is considered mere fluff and a financial burden on for-profit hospitals. Hospital chaplains' pay—if they are lucky enough to land positions— is abominable. Many hospitals either have furloughed chaplains—as the pandemic is costing hospitals too much money—or hospital administrators are simply getting rid of chaplains altogether. Chaplains do not generate income. What generates income—in for-profit hospitals—means leaner staff. Hospital chaplains are seen as in the way, extra, not meaningful—because they do not generate capital. The lack of trained chaplains in hospitals does a great disservice not only to patients but to hospital staff as well. The lack of trained hospital chaplains—as Boisen knew so well from first-hand experience—does violence to those who need emotional and spiritual support the most. During the pandemic families are desperate and have no one to turn to except chaplains. Nurses and doctors are not trained to deal with emotions and spiritual issues with which that families are dealing. The erasure of the human and humane from medical treatment was exactly why Boisen (1952) began the field of hospital chaplaincy to begin with. The erasure of chaplaincy in for-profit hospitals is a political and curricular matter. We see similar trends in the academy as humanities are being cut, philosophy departments are closing, and theology is disappearing with the exception of work being done in seminaries. However, seminaries are not universities.

Boisen's (1952) dream, at one time, played an important role in hospital curriculum and the medical humanities. But today, all of that is changing. I do not know what future there is in hospital chaplaincy, if there is a future at all. The same could be said about the humanities in the university. Do the humanities have a future at all?

Louise DeSalvo: An Unbearable Story Etched in Memory-Traces

Louise DeSalvo (2018) in her memoirs *The House of Early Sorrows* reminds that abusive childhood marks a life forever. Like Derrick Jensen (2000)—who suffered a horrific childhood because of his father's violence—Louise DeSalvo suffered from growing up in a violent home as well, never seeming to get peace from her memories, although she states that writing helps her cope. It is interesting that both Jensen (2000) and DeSalvo (2018) became writers. Writing as a coping mechanism is what Freud recommended to his patients who suffered childhood trauma. Writing does not always heal old wounds. Sometimes, in fact, writing serves to re-traumatize and can make things worse.

DeSalvo (1980) is known mostly for her biography of Virginia Woolf. DeSalvo states that there is a connection between her work on Woolf and her own family disasters.

> I wonder whether I have chosen to work on Virginia Woolf because of the similarities between her family's history and my own. In making out a work plan when I return home... I write, "Think about [Virginia]Woolf again. (Six years later, I publish a book-length study about Woolf as an incest survivor. (1980. p. 112)

DeSalvo tells her readers that she too was a victim of incest. Nietzsche once remarked that we look for people who are like ourselves in what we read. In the case of DeSalvo, Freud might suggest that her work on Virginia Woolf makes sense because we do what is familiar, we write about what we know, whether we are aware of it or not. Woolf's situation was a familiar one for DeSalvo.

DeSalvo reports that she not only suffered from childhood incest, she suffered from the violence of her parent's rage. Her father tried to kill her with a butcher knife, the very knife her mother used in the kitchen; the very knife that was the symbol of her mother's rage as well. The family romance, as Freud called it, is the scene of cruelty, the scene of violence. Incest is not romance—and certainly Freud did not mean it that way—incest is violence, just as the family romance is violent. Freud suggested that there is, in fact, no romance in the family at all. The family is the site of Oedipal violence.

DeSalvo (2018) and Jensen (2000) share many of the same kinds of violent experiences as children. Although both of these writers differ from one another in many ways; it is the very act of writing that seems to sustain them. DeSalvo wanted so to understand her childhood that she attempted to corroborate her recollections with her siblings. But she said that this became a problem because no one wanted to talk; curiously, no one seemed to remember anything. DeSalvo (2018) asks

> How to you tell the story of a people who don't want to remember, who don't often tell you what they recall or, if they do they speak in puzzles, riddles, enigmas.... Because the stories people try to forget are the most important stories, the ones that must be recorded, the ones history has buried or ignored or erased, the one memoirists must tell. Memoir, then, is a corrective to history. (p. xvi)

DeSalvo (2018) resonates with Freud's basic premise that when in analysis, the analysand's silences tell the tale more so than what is directly spoken. It is the not-said that matters most, Freud stressed. But as DeSalvo (2018) asks: Is it not important, too, to get at what is not said. Memoirs are relational; one does not remember things in a vacuum, and others are always already implicated and or embroiled. The story one tells about one's own life is also the story that also includes the lives of others. Whether those other stories are directly told or not: they hover in the background. However, when others, as DeSalvo (2018) reports, either cannot remember much or refuse to tell what they do remember memoir work becomes more difficult. The very act of memoir writing becomes haunted by ghosts, or specters, by the stories that have been deliberately withheld, or unconsciously forgotten as memory traces. Derrida (1994) states

> If I am getting ready to speak at length about ghosts, inheritance, and generations, and generations of ghosts, which is to say about certain others who are not present, not presently living, either to us, in us, or outside us, it is in the name of justice. (p. xix)

DeSalvo (2018) writes about generations of her own family members who suffered from either alcoholism, or abuse partly because of ongoing discrimination against Italians and Italian Americans—as her family came from Italy. When a family is treated less than human upon arrival to the shores of another country—as were many Italians upon their arrival to the United States during the turn of the 20th century—the psychological turning against the self, as Freud would call it, plays out as internalized self-hatred and violence projected onto others. DeSalvo suggests that the generations of Italians who immigrated to the United States suffered perhaps a worse fate here than in Italy. This point, too, was made by Upton Sinclair (2006) in *The Jungle*, as he suggested that Lithuanian immigrants suffered a worse fate in the United States than they did back home.

The meat packing industry treated immigrants inhumanely, to say the least. In fact, conditions in the meat packing industry in Chicago were so horrific—and Sinclair's book made such an impact on President Teddy Roosevelt that he initiated the FDA in order to regulate meat packing factories in the attempt to make these kinds of industries safer and more humane places.

Like the horrible plight of the Lithuanian immigrants, Sinclair brought to light, DeSalvo (2018) writes about the sufferings of Italian American immigrants. Curriculum theorist Paula Salvio (2017), likewise, has written an important work on the ongoing problem of discrimination against Italian Americans. The TV show, *The Sopranos*, a popular HBO series—that ran for years, until about 2007—about an Italian Mafia family in New Jersey —(which is still popular among young people today perhaps because the Sopranos serves as an escapist fantasy of gang-life for many who feel isolated during the pandemic) probably fed the stereotype that all Italians are in the Mafia. *The Sopranos*—although based on a true story of a Mafia family from New Jersey—has actually done a great disservice to the Italian American community—by (perhaps unwittingly) perpetuating stereotypes about the Italian American community.

DeSalvo (2018) writes about how difficult it was for her family to immigrate from Sicily to the United States. She tells us about her grandmother who refused to wear anything other than black clothes—as a symbol of Italian identity, or perhaps as a symbol of perpetual mourning of a lost identity and culture. As a child, DeSalvo (2018) stated that her grandmother embarrassed her because she refused to assimilate into American culture. The refusal to wear anything but black was perhaps symbolic of her refusal to assimilate. Despite being embarrassed by her grandmother's appearance, DeSalvo admits that it was her grandmother who stepped between her father and the butcher knife he wielded at DeSalvo, even as a child. It was her grandmother—the woman who refused to dress in anything but black—who literally saved her life numerous times from being stabbed to death.

DeSalvo (2018) also writes about the regrets and confusions she had about her mother especially when she became ill and died. DeSalvo (2018) states that although she wanted to love her mother she knew she did not, she could not, and yet she had regrets that she did not. This is a very difficult thing to admit in a culture that honors the Ten Commandments, one of which is honor thy mother and thy father. Therapist Alice Miller (2001) states that the majority of her patients suffered from honoring this commandment because it was drilled into them as children; those who honored their mother and father—no matter what—suffered the most from guilt and depression because they could not manage their mangled and conflicting emotions, especially if they were abused by their parents.

Like Derrick Jensen (2000), DeSalvo writes in order to tell the truth; to find, perhaps some kind of solace from telling the truth, and maybe even as Derrida puts it, to find "justice" (1994, p. xix). Unlike Jensen (2000), DeSalvo wrote her memoir after her entire family died. Jensen did not wait until his father died to tell the tale. It is a precarious decision to make to write horror stories about one's parents when they are still alive.

As the pandemic rages on into its third year and the variants get more and more dangerous, domestic abuse and violence keep ticking upwards as I mentioned earlier. Families are stretched to their breaking points. Teachers and students are forced to go back into the classrooms in dangerous, precarious situations. The omicron and deltacron variants are highly transmissible and are wreaking havoc among school children, their parents, the teachers and putting enormous strain on hospital systems that are nearing collapse. Republican governors and state legislatures continue on with their do-nothing policies, and now children and young people are dying in overflowing hospitals with fewer and fewer ICU beds. Health care professionals are exhausted. Teachers are exhausted and the worry seems never to end. These stressors result in anger, rage and violence. Pent up hostilities are the quickest way to release rage. Hospitals are not only seeing dramatic rises in covid cases—with bad outcomes, even for young children—but the uptick in gun violence, stabbings, car accidents caused by road rage, suicides and utter hopelessness, confusion and denial.

Once hospitalized, if patients survive, at least in the United States, they cannot pay their medical bills and are forced into bankruptcy. People are losing their homes, they cannot pay their rent; people are getting evicted. Inflation is at a forty-year high, the economy is teetering on the edge, everything seems as if it is spiraling out of control.

There seems no end to these unbearable stories. I have called the ongoing violence, rage and domestic violence covid collateral (Morris, 2021a). Although DeSalvo's (2018) and Jensen's (2000) memoirs were written before the advent of covid, their stories are not unfamiliar and, in fact, stories of abuse—like theirs—have only intensified because of covid. Utter frustration on the part of teachers, faculty members at universities and colleges—who are not unionized—are scared and helpless. Mbembe's (2019) work on what he calls *Necropolitics* –the politics of death in its interconnection with racism and health care—is real. Those whose lives do not seem to matter, people of color, the poor, those without money or health insurance who have no hope for a future, have no future. Who survives? Who decides? When ICU beds run out—even at children's hospitals (in pediatric intensive care units)—who lives and who dies? Although it is illegal to engage in what is called patient dumping—a practice whereby emergency rooms refuse treatment to those who cannot pay—there are other ways of not providing services after the emergency room visit, that are legal. Those without the capital, do not benefit from the best therapies, because those are reserved for the wealthy. When there are no more beds in ICUs patients will have to be turned away and die at home, or die on the streets.

It is important to document social and political events—as Hannah Arendt (1979; 1994; 2003; 2005) pointed out decades ago. Being an academic does not mean that one is sheltered from the storm; in fact, academics should be in the middle of the storm. Intellectuals' first responsibility is to public service and to public intellectual work. As obscure and abstract as intellectual work can become, it can also put those abstractions to work for the public good. This is the meaning of the public intellectual. Edward Said (1996) states: "There is no such thing as a private intellectual, since the moment you set down words and then publish them you have entered the public world" (p. 12). Bertrand Russell most noted for his work in mathematical logic and analytic philosophy is one of the few analytic philosophers who engaged in the work of the public intellectual. Peter Stone (2016) suggests that although Russell was not considered a political philosopher—say in the tradition of Hannah Arendt or Noam Chomsky—still he engaged in writing about politics. Stone (2016) tells us that Russell "described himself as writing about politics merely as a concerned human being, but this may indeed be too modest a characterization after all…. Alan Ryan describes Russell as a political polemicist, a pamphleteer in the tradition of Thomas Paine" (p. 129).

It is curious why it is that politics fell out of fashion for philosophers given that the ancient Greek word *Agora* means to gather or to assemble in the public to discuss political and philosophical issues. Is this not what Socrates did? His work was public; he worked in the street and asked people to tell him about their lives. Of course, there was more to it than that as Socrates did have an agenda: to get people to better understand their tasks in life and to better take care of themselves. But interestingly he did not consider himself a teacher. He felt that the knowledge people had was already within them. He served as a midwife to knowledge. And he annoyed people as well: the Gadfly is what Socrates was called. Socrates annoyed people because he told people things that they did not want to hear. Socrates attempted to get people to understand that they did not understand what they thought they did and perhaps their arrogance and self-flattery got in the way of their understanding. In that tradition, Edward Said (1996) states: "Least of all should an intellectual be there to make his/her audience feel good: the whole point is to be embarrassing, contrary, and even unpleasant"

(p. 12). Foucault (2011) points out in his last lectures *The Courage of Truth*, that many ancient Greek philosophers frowned on those who were ingratiating; those were the ones who were called flatterers. And to be called a flatterer was an insult.

The problem with the modern university—which is hardly an *Agora*—is that flattery is encouraged; being a gadfly is not. One of the ways professors survive in universities is through flattery and ingratiating behavior. There is little room for dissensus; little tolerance for true debate. If one dares to have the "courage" to tell the truth—to be a risk taker—as Foucault (2011) argues that we should—one also risks not getting tenure, or not being promoted. Socrates risked death. And Socrates accepted his fate—as unjust as it was—because he risked his life in order to be a truth-teller. Socrates he had the *courage* to speak truth to power. For Foucault (2011) it is the courage to be a truth-teller, to speak truth to power—despite the consequences—that makes for the true philosopher. Being a professional philosopher—today—does not necessarily mean that one is a true philosopher in the sense that Socrates meant it. If one is not willing to risk everything for the sake of truth; if one is not willing to risk death for the sake of truth one is not a true philosopher but a mere sophist.

What is striking in the memoirs I have written about here—for Boisen (1958), Jensen (2000) and DeSalvo (2018) is that they are not only personal but they are also political. All three memoirs are commentaries on the cruelties of violence and the ethical obligation to right was is wrong through the very act of writing. All three of these memoirists demonstrate the courage to speak truth to power. Telling unbearable stories—in these particular cases—are not merely self-serving or narcissistic. The personal is political, as feminists have pointed out long ago. But still, some political scholars see little point in personal story telling; however, these their criticisms are unfounded. The socio-political is inextricably tied to the personal.

The greater problem is not speaking truth to power. And as I have written elsewhere (Morris 2021b), the entire history of *Bildung* in the Germanic philosophic tradition is guilty of turning away from the political. This apolitical ideology leads straight to fascism and totalitarianism. Kierkegaard's notion that truth is subjectivity is only half true. Yes, truth is subjectivity but only when one is socially and politically engaged. George Herbert Mead long ago taught that the self is social. That truth is subjectivity in the context of the socio-political, that the self is only a self in relation to the Other avoids the problems of solipsism and self-preoccupation. To pretend that one does not have to be concerned about the larger socio-political world is a recipe for disaster.

John Gunther

John Gunther's (1949) memoir about his teenage son's death from a brain tumor leaves one aghast. This is a story that certainly leaves the reader "undone" (Butler, 2019, p. 136). Judith Butler states: "To be undone by another is a primary necessity, an anguish, to be sure, but also to be moved, to be prompted to act" (p. 136). If one is not ready to be "undone" one should not attempt to read Gunther's memoir. This is a gut-wrenching story that is almost too much to bear. Perhaps the agony of Gunther's story is due to the fact that it concerns a young person—a teenager—who dies a horrific death. I have worked in pediatric ICUs and have witnessed the cruel deaths of children. As a chaplain I have been called in to be with parents who suffer the deaths of their children from drownings, gun shot wounds, illnesses beyond description. There is nothing more difficult for a chaplain—at least in my experience—than being called to the pediatric ICU or the children's hospital.

To be there with the physician when the bad news is broken to the parents is the worst part of the job. After the physician leaves the room, the chaplain is there to pick up the pieces of broken lives. But picking up the pieces of broken lives is impossible when it comes to the deaths of children and young people. The parents who are so distraught, most in disbelief or denial; sometimes totally overcome by grief or shock, have only the company of the chaplain after the physician leaves the room. And for some, even the company of the chaplain is too much. On many occasions, I have been asked to leave. Parents want to grieve alone.

There is no company—so to speak—in the face of the death of a child. Parents often ask the question why. How could it be that a child has died? The chaplain has no answers. All chaplains can offer is their presence. There is nothing to say. Consolations only make things worse.

John Gunther (1949) writes about his teenage son, Johnny, who dies of a brain tumor. The story sweeps the reader away in the quickness of the events that unfold and Johnny's untimely ending. Gunther ends the story by telling us that he "felt his [Johnny's] arms, cupping my hands around them, and the warmth gradually left them., receding very slowly upward from his hands. For a long time some warmth remained. Then little by little the life-color left his face, his lips became blue, and his hands were cold. What is life? It departs covertly. Like a thief Death took him" (p. 137). As a chaplain I have witnessed thousands of patients die. And Gunther's description of death is the way I have seen it unfold too. Eventually the body turns blue, eventually the body grows cold. But what eventually happens—the body turning blue and cold—happens rather quickly. It is alarming how quickly life disappears. What one does with that disappearance emotionally I do not know.

Throughout Gunther's (1949) memoir he struggles whether to tell his son the truth about his tumor or not. He opts not to tell him the truth. It is a truth that he thinks is just too unbearable, perhaps for himself as well as for his son. Gunther (1949) states:

> Of course Johnny did not know the full seriousness of his illness. Above all we had to shield him from the difficult, explicit knowledge, since his greatest asset by far—his only asset aside from his youth—was his will to live. (pp. 38-39)

To tell the truth or not. This is a problem with which bioethicists wrestle. Those in the medical profession know that in the 1940s it was common not to tell patients the truth; this was common medical practice. Physicians felt that it was only cruelty to tell the truth; in Johnny's case it would be better in the long run not to tell him the truth, or so they thought. However, this practice of doctors not telling patients the truth has changed. I have heard doctors tell families the truth—in the most blunt, brutal ways. I often wonder if they think they are doing the families a service by being blunt. Some doctors, however, have more tact than others and are quite gentle when breaking bad news to families. Doctors are supposed to tell the truth to their patients and their families, but on occasion I have heard doctors lie, especially in the emergency room. The rules of etiquette in the emergency room are different than in an ICU. If doctors tell patients the truth, they could go into shock. So even though medical ethics prohibits lying to patients, doctors do it anyway when they feel that it might do more harm than good.

Foucault (2011) writes about what he calls a "crisis of *parrhesia*" (p. 35). *Parrhesia* is the Greek word for truth. Foucault tells us that this "crisis... appears in the philosophical and political literature of the fourth century" (p. 35). But this crisis has nothing to do with whether or not to tell a person that they are facing death. The crisis to which Foucault speaks concerns truth-telling in a democracy where anybody is allowed to say anything; the crisis of truth-telling in a democracy, Foucault argues is that anybody can say anything—and that is a problem. Anything can be truth for anyone. This radical relativism can be very dangerous. Who decides what truth is if anybody can say anything? This is why the ancient Greek philosophers—like Plato—did not feel that democracy was the best form of government. Rather, Plato preferred monarchy because the truth could be contained. Truth-tellers, for Plato, were philosophers-kings. They are the only ones who are the guardians of truth; because they are wise enough to know the difference between truth and lies. That the Republic must be governed by philosopher-kings, or at least become advisors to princes or other figures of a monarchy, meant that the Republic would be protected from those who would say anything, or even lie. Philosopher-kings knew enough to avoid tyranny. If anybody can say anything—in a democratic form of government—that means anything goes. Radical relativism leads to the utter collapse of a republic.

The crisis of truth in a medical setting, however, differs from the problems that occupied ancient Greek philosophers. The crisis of truth-telling when a child is dying brings with it its own set of serious dilemmas. What do parents do? What is the ethical obligation to truth-telling on the part of medical personnel? Wilder Penfield—one of Johnny's physicians—decided that to be blunt and brutally honest was the only choice he had when speaking with Gunther. Penfield, however, did not break this brutal news to Johnny—who was but a teenager. Gunther (1949) states "Penfield cut through all the euphemisms and said directly, 'Your child has a malignant glioma, and it will kill him'" (p. 55).

I suppose it is one thing to tell the brutal honest truth to a parent of a dying child, but another thing to tell the child—at least in that manner. I have heard some pediatricians tell parents after a child dies, her siblings should be told the truth. But how? When? And then what? A woman who lost her child to covid had four other small children. These children could not have been more than five years old or so. When the children came into the trauma bay—not a common practice—they had no idea what was going on. In fact, the children tried to console their mother, saying, don't cry mama, it's okay. The children did not understand what had happened, even though they saw the dead child in their mother's arms. This was a heartbreaking scene.

Johnny, Gunther's son, did not have siblings—at least none were mentioned in the book. Still, Gunther grappled with what to say and what not to say. Gunther does admit toward the end of the memoir that perhaps he should have told Johnny the truth because keeping up the façade and all the lies only exhausted Johnny more. In the end, Johnny intuited that he was dying anyway. However, Gunther (1949) confesses that "[o]ver and over we told Johnny, lying, that the tumor was dead, that Putnam [the surgeon] *had* [italics in the original] got it all" (p. 42). Unlike the story told by Terry Tempest Williams (2001) in *Refuge*, although her mother was dying of cancer, too—albeit of a wholly different kind—Williams' mother was an adult, not a child. In the case of a child dying or a young person—a teenager—truth-telling becomes a crisis and an ethical dilemma.

Derrida (2001) asks: "Over what are we keeping watch? Are we trying to negate death or retain it" (p. 50)? Of course, no one wants to witness the death of one's child. No one wants to admit that children can, indeed, pre-decease their parents. But the "negation" of death is magical thinking. On one level, it is clear that Gunther (1949) did not, in fact, negate the death of his son, or engage in magical thinking. However, on another level, one might wonder what the title of his memoir really means. *Death Be Not Proud* the title of Gunther's memoir is based on the well-known poem by John Donne.

This poem is difficult to understand in and of itself; it is also difficult to understand why this poem would be the title of Gunther's memoir because he seemed to accept the death of his son and not engage in magical thinking. However, the poem *Death Be Not Proud* is the Christian antidote to death, and it is, indeed, magical thinking. The line "death be not proud" means there is no death. The afterlife is after death and this, therefore, "negates" death, to draw on Derrida (2001, p. 50).

The majority of Christians I have worked with as a chaplain in the hospital believe in life after death and often say—after the death of a child—he will no longer suffer, he is going to a better place. Or they will resort to it is God's will that their child died; God's will be done, they say, reciting a line from the Bible. But what kind of a God wills the death of a child?

Michel Serres (2001) writes about the ancient poet Lucretius' view of death. According to Serres (2001), Lucretius felt that "[t]he world, objects, bodies... from the time of their birth [are] adrift.... This means, in common terms, that they [bodies] irreversibly fall apart and die" (p. 50). That sentient beings are "adrift" and bound to die is a thought with which most grapple. But a 17 year old—like Gunther's son Johnny—does not usually think about death. Isn't it rather cruel that someone that young "irreversibly fall[s] apart and die[s]" (Lucretius, cited in Serres, 2001, p. 50)? Whether one faces the ruthless truth of dying—in these terms—or engages in magical thinking that life after death negates death, either way, the cold hard truth of the matter, or consolations through magical thinking, still do not make things any easier in the end. Not that one should engage in consolation, but the question is how does one cope with one's mortality at all, especially as a teenager?

The opening line of Gunther's (1949) memoir somehow does not sit right. Gunther states (1949) "*This is not so much a memoir of Johnny in the conventional sense* as the story of a long, courageous struggle between a child and death" (p. 3). What is, in fact, "courageous" about knowing one is about to die? Foucault (2011) uses the term courage as one makes a conscious decision to risk truth-telling.

Aristotle (1987), in *The Nichomachean Ethics* writes about courage as a virtue. But in the face of death—especially the death of a child or a young person—the word courage makes little sense. When people have said to me, for example, you have handled your cancer diagnosis courageously I cringe because I know that courage has had little to do with handling a cancer diagnosis. Courage and virtue have little to do with coping with a cancer diagnosis. Somehow these words seem antiquated, idealistic and out of touch with the reality at hand. The term courage, like bravery, simply do not make sense in these contexts. These words might be better suited for soldiers who have been in combat. But living with cancer or dying from cancer is not a form of combat. Susan Gubar (2012) suggests that military metaphors—around cancer—are highly problematic. Gubar asks: what if you die from cancer? Are you then a loser? Losing a battle with cancer also suggests that you were simply not strong enough to fight it. But the unwieldy replication of cells within one's body cannot be fought the way a war is fought. Moreover, military metaphors—often unthought—mean that only the winners get to tell their stories. Nobody wants to hear the stories of losers. One of the reasons that there are not many narratives on ovarian cancer—Gubar (2012) suggests—is that first off, most women with ovarian cancer die and do not have the time to write a memoir, and secondly nobody wants to hear the story of losers. Dying from cancer is not something people want to read about. People want to read narratives of survival, not death. In battle, the winners are glorified; the losers are forgotten in the ashbins of history. But cancer is neither a battle, nor a war. There are no winners and losers in the context of cancer. And certainly being courageous has little to do with the life and death of someone who succumbs to cancer. It is not a virtue to live or die from cancer. It is not a virtue to be stoic in the face of cancer. Cancer has nothing to do with virtue or courage. Living or dying from cancer is a nightmare: it is an unbearable story.

Cancer patients and those who are undergoing chemotherapy are more vulnerable to infections because they are immune-suppressed. In the context of covid, having cancer or having had chemotherapy can be quite frightening in the age of covid. When one is immune-compromised, the chances of getting very ill from covid are higher than if one is not immune-compromised.

Of course, Gunther's (1949) memoir has nothing to do with covid. However, his memoir is relevant—in today's context—on many levels. As was mentioned earlier, going into the third year of the pandemic the delta variant, the omicron and deltacron variants and perhaps those that are to follow—because there will be more of them—are making children very ill. In fact, some children are dying from covid. The situation is made worse when a child is also suffering from cancer, undergoing chemotherapy and is immune-compromised. Children who have had cancer have little protection against covid and if they contract covid, suffering from co-morbidities makes life all the more precarious.

There is not much discussion currently about childhood cancer in collision with covid. There is not much discussion currently about any childhood diseases in collision with covid. There are many diseases that bring about immune-compromised situations. Chemotherapy basically destroys the immune system and its long-term effects are not really known. It used to be thought that the effects of chemotherapy wore off after some time. But that is not always the case. Chemotherapy can leave one immune-compromised for a very long time. Chemotherapy can cause nerve disorders decades later; secondary cancers from chemotherapy can emerge decades after having had chemotherapy. Chemotherapy causes brain fog—as does covid—and this might not be temporary for some. The collision of covid and chemotherapy for those who already suffer from brain fog devastates. The exhaustion from chemotherapy is long lasting and in collision with covid—which is also exhausting—disastrous effects can ensue. Gunther's (1949) memoir still resonates today. People still lose their children to cancer and other horrible diseases. Children who are now dying of covid, may be perfectly healthy otherwise. Or, children who die from covid might suffer co-morbidities like cancer.

Covid deaths are often reduced to numbers on TV. Deaths reduced to numbers is another way to erase and whitewash the archive of covid. Judith Butler (2016) points out that "[w]e read about lives lost and are often given the numbers, but these stories are repeated every day, and the repetition appears endless, irremediable" (p. 13). The ongoing tallies we see on TV every night become numbing and meaningless after a while. Lives reduced to numbers serve to numb. The continual tallying of meaningless numbers of covid deaths on TV serves to desensitize. After a while, the psyche cannot process these numbers. And this, too, is what happens to frontline workers in health care settings.

After a while, the covid numbers climb while the deaths from covid have become almost routinized. Medical professionals know that this is what happens when confronting so much trauma. But without psychological defense mechanisms, such as numbing, medical personnel could not function at all. The problems begin when the defense mechanisms get in the way of living a life, get in the way of feeling anything at all. After this nightmare of covid is over, will medical personnel become ghosts to themselves? Derrida (1994)—in the context of Marx—writes about specters, ghosts, *revenants*, as was mentioned earlier in this chapter. Will we all become ghosts to ourselves after this nightmare is over? Or will this nightmare never end? How will we survive these unbearable stories, if we survive at all?

7

Albert Camus' Relevance for Unbearable Stories of the Covid Pandemic

In order to better understand Camus' overarching philosophical stance, it is necessary to deconstruct his work against the backdrop of his biographic situation. I have always found Camus difficult to untangle, let alone understand. This chapter will be a labyrinthine archivization of Camus' oeuvre in the context of his life story in order that we may better understand Camus' (1948) novel *The Plague* and why this book, in particular, is so relevant to today's covid pandemic in the intersection of the trend toward authoritarianism in the United States.

Olivier Todd (2000) claims that although Camus stated that "A man's works often describe his longings or temptations… almost never his own true story"… [Camus's work] "is highly autobiographical" (Todd, 2000, p. x). That writings are shot through with "longings and temptations" does not make them any less important. Autobiographical writing is never truth with a capital T, nor is biography. But getting at the Truth with a capital T is not the point.

Jacques Derrida (1991) further complicates the issue by contending that the original meaning of a text is altered by the reader's interpretation. Derrida (1991) says about reading and writing that

> For all these quotations, quotations of requotations with no original performance, there is no speech act not already the iteration of another, no circle and

no quotation marks to reassure us about the identity, opposition, or distinction of speech events. (p. 263)

In other words, Derrida suggests that texts are always already read out of context. Interpretation of texts alter the original intent of the author. Hence, the reader's perspective on Camus and the context in which the reader interprets Camus makes way for a different "iteration" altering the original intention.

The Life and the Work: Philosophers in Context

To put a philosopher's work in context means to place his/her work against the backdrop of a life story. Not all philosophers agree that this is important or necessary. But if readers want to better understand the texts that come before them, it is important to know something about the person who wrote the texts that they are studying. Psycho-biographies—psychoanalyzing someone's biography—have long fallen out of fashion; historians squashed the discipline of psycho-biography long ago. Historians are suspicious of psychoanalytic theory in the context of historiography. Historians are empiricists. Certainly, though, there are other ways of reading texts: strict empirical methodology stifles. Perhaps psychoanalytic theory (rather than strict empiricism) might open pathways that are unthought that help readers understand who it is that they are reading in the first place.

Jacques Derrida in the film *Derrida* (2003) contends that in the context of philosophy and biography there are two words that philosophers might ruminate upon. Derrida asks that philosophers consider "*The Who"* and "*The What*"—philosophically. The Who—refers to the writer who writes the text at hand. The What—refers to the text. "*The Who and The What*", Derrida argues, cannot be separated. Who writes what matters. Yet, traditionally—Derrida (2003) points out—philosophers have had little interest in the *who*. Part of the problem is that life stories muddy the water of the texts which philosophers write. Ruth Behar (1997) points out that George Devereux once stated that methods used generally in the social sciences—or I might add in the humanities as well-"'reduce anxiety and enable us to function efficiently' (cited in Behar, p. 6) or, in another way, Devereaux puts it, methodologies are used to 'drain anxiety'" (p. 6). Historians—and perhaps philosophers—are notably afraid of writing through their own emotions; in fact, they are taught methodologically, to erase their emotions and rely on clear and straight forward language. A curriculum that dives into anxiety, rather than draining it, is especially relevant to the ways in which Camus' work helps to us to make connections to our current covid catastrophe.

Historians have long argued that you cannot psychoanalyze the dead. This writer asks: why not? Psychoanalytic theory is metaphor; psychoanalytic theory is not about getting at empirical truth, it never was—even as Freud conceptualized it. Recall, Freud drew on Greek mythology to come to ideas about subjectivity. Freud was not interested in literal truth(s). Like Freud, Camus (1955/1983) points out that at the end of the day, "a man [sic] remains forever unknown to us… there is something irreducible that escapes us" (p. 11). Although we "remain" *strangers*—as Camus might put it—to one another, still some psychological insight into another can be gleaned. And from that insight, philosophical questions might arise.

It is the case that philosophers and psychoanalysts' disciplines could not be more different. Philosophers are mostly interested in what is conscious while psychoanalysts are interested in what is unconscious. Yet, it is precisely this difference (between these disciplines) that might make a difference—as Gregory Bateson (2000) would put it—in the ways philosophical horizons open anew.

For Freud, what matters most especially in childhood—and throughout adult life as well—are the little things ignored or forgotten. Freud, much like a detective, looked for the little—and seemingly insignificant things—that tend to get ignored, when attempting to uncover a life. Following Freud, this chapter focuses on some seemingly insignificant moments from Camus's childhood through a psychoanalytic lens in order to attempt to unpack Camus's work in "a new key," (Langer, 1957).

Childhood during the covid crisis is especially difficult. Children—whether they attend school or do remote learning—are living through an historical catastrophe. Isolation, distance and coping with the death of people around them—perhaps even their parents or siblings—is too much to bear. Camus' childhood was a troubled one. Some of Camus' issues arose from the feelings of isolation, distance and coping with emotional turmoil from his father's death to his mother's muteness and her emotional distance. What we learn from Camus' experiences can connect—in metaphoric ways—to what it is that children are experiencing now during the covid crisis. This is what I call a curriculum of metaphor through literary fiction.

Camus' (1995) fictionized childhood in *The First Man* matters. *The First Man* was actually the last book that Camus wrote. The manuscript was found in the trunk of a car, after a terrible accident in which Camus was killed. He never saw the manuscript through to publication. His wife did not want the manuscript published. After she died, Camus's daughter Catherine—in consultation with her brother—decided to publish the manuscript as is. Although Catherine Camus (1995) tells us that she thought that her father would have probably edited the manuscript while he was alive, she and her brother did not want editors to alter it posthumously. The manuscript was penned in 1960 but was not published until 1995.

The most stunning passage in *The First Man* concerns his partially deaf mother—who is fictionalized in the text—over whom he both loved and anguished. Camus's mother

> then assumed once more her motionless position, in the shadow half-light, her gaze lost in the street and the current of life that flowed endlessly below the riverbank where she sat endlessly, while her son, endlessly, watched her in the shadows with a lump in his throat... filled with an obscure anxiety in the presence of adversity he could not understand. (Camus, 1995, p. 228)

Notably, the word "endlessly" is repeated three times in this short passage. Camus's mother's life was "endlessly" about nothing. This "endless" nothingness is painful to read. Imagine a life of "endless" nothingness. The "motionless[ness]" and the lost "gaze" marks an emotional state of withdrawal and distance. During the covid crisis, as a chaplain I have witnessed those who—in the beginning of the pandemic—were allowed to visit their dying loved ones and stare through glass-enclosed rooms to say their last goodbyes—also exhibited a kind of "motionless" lost "gaze" while in disbelief at their loved one dying hooked up to machines and unconscious.

The "endless" nothing of living without meaning was partly due to Camus' mother being "partially deaf", and emotionally stultified. Sometimes Camus' mother spoke but what she understood is not known fully. Olivier Todd (2000) states that Catherine Helene Sintes-Camus was

> Partly deaf, she could neither read nor write. Although she was able to read lips some people thought her mute, or mentally retarded. Others thought that she was suffering from badly treated meningitis. Albert believed that his mother began to have hearing and speech problems after a bout of typhoid fever or typhus. Still others thought she had had a cerebral attack upon hearing about her husband's death. (p. 7).

Camus's mother could not understand much, she could not read, she did not ask "Jacques" (Camus' pseudonym in *The First Man*) much. Camus seemed to have an unconscious—or perhaps conscious—bond with his mother throughout his life. One wonders whether the "lump in his (Jacques') throat" is what drove Camus to become a philosopher. That lump signifies a heartache so deep that no words could express his sorrow and anguish. Much of Camus' fiction anguishes; much of Camus' fiction was philosophical and stressed emotional states beyond signification.

Even though *The First Man* is partly a story about Camus' birthing himself without a father—because he was killed in WW1 while Camus was an infant—it seems that his anguished relationship with his mother takes center stage. But still the search for the absent father haunted Camus. Camus' anguish over his mother and longing for his absent father—informs mostly all of his work in one way or another. Herbert Lottman (1997) comments:

> When Albert Camus spoke of his father it was necessarily at a remove, for no articulate witness, scarcely a document, survived to bridge the bottomless chasm separating a father who died after wounds received in the Battle of the Marne and an infant less than a year old when it happened. (p. 14)

Jacques—the pseudonym for Camus in *The First Man*—feels that his father—who was killed in the Great War—died a "stranger" (p. 27) to the world: "no one had known him but his mother and she had forgotten him" (p. 27). Perhaps Camus felt a moral obligation to pay respects to his dead and forgotten father. Oddly, the visit to his father's grave psychically and metaphorically resurrects his father. "His father was alive again, a strange silent life" (p. 28). And yet his father was dead.

Like Camus' father's ghostly presence after his death, Camus seemed haunted—as well—by his mother's silence and indifference. Was she psychically dead to him too—yet ghostly alive? Could it be that the "dead mother syndrome"—as psychoanalyst Andre Green (1993) calls it—applied both to his mother and his father? Green explains that the "dead mother syndrome" is metaphorical—that the mother, or primary figure—becomes psychically dead to the child—even if the primary figure is alive. One might also apply this theory to primal figures who are dead—even though this is not Green's (1993) meaning. Psychoanalysts Nicholas Abraham and Maria Torok (1978) introduced the notion of a psychic "phantom" that haunts victims of trauma—even transgenerationally. For Abraham and Torok (1978) whether primal figures are dead or alive, whether stories (of trauma) are told or not, psychic ghosts take up inhabitance in a "crypt" in the psyche. Psychic "phantoms" take on a life of their own—especially if trauma cannot be consciously articulated. Ironically—especially in the cases of traumatic death—the longer a primal figure is dead—the more alive—in the psyche—that primal figure—becomes. One wonders, then, to what extent, Camus felt tormented—or perhaps haunted and abandoned—by his dead and ghostly father and his ghost-like mother.

One might wonder how the transgenerational trauma of the covid pandemic will affect children who have lost their parents to this virus. What "phantoms" will they hand down to their children and the next generation after that? An entire generation of children will suffer some kind of psychic trauma because of this pandemic. How are we to educate an entire generation of traumatized children? Melanie Klein (1992)—who was the first psychoanalyst to work with children in the early 1920s—suggested that very young children play with dolls and toys. In that play, children would act out the emotions that they are feeling, since they might not yet be able to verbalize them. The psychoanalytic approach to trauma—like the approach that chaplains use with patients who have been traumatized—is to allow pain, suffering, anguish to be expressed. No false hope, no consolations, no toxic positivity. The psychoanalytic model, it must be noted, is the exact opposite of the model used by social workers, who work from peoples' strengths and give the hope that the future will be better. But this is not what chaplains or psychoanalysts do—because the future might not be better, false hope is dangerous and working from strengths is unrealistic when a mother loses a child, or a child loses a mother.

Jacques in *The First Man*—felt that it was not his father who had abandoned him during the war, but that he himself had "abandoned" (p. 28) his father as he "turn[ed} "his back on the grave" (1995, p. 28). Perhaps this psychological reversal—of who abandoned whom—was a result of survivor's guilt and the inability to emotionally negotiate his father's death. Camus was very young when his father was killed.

Ironically, the less one knows about a primal figure's death, the more intense the fantasies—about that death—become. Freud argued that reality—indeed—is shot through with fantasy. But in the case of experiencing the death of a parent, these fantasies can torment. Children especially have vivid imaginations which might turn into vivid nightmares or night terrors, even if they know little about their parent's death.

Melanie Klein (1993) suggested that infants' destructive phantasies dominate their psychic world. In the preverbal stage, Klein wrote that infants feel threatened by "persecutory" (p. 2) anxiety (by the phantasy that mother will kill them). Consequently, infants have a fear of suffering "annihilation" (p. 4). Klein emphasizes that these kinds of phantasies are driven by paranoia. This, Klein called the paranoid-schizoid phase. As the infant matures, however, guilt and reparation (called the depressive phase) emerge (Klein, 1992). Those who do not work through the depressive phase—risk becoming paranoid-schizophrenics, or perhaps even sociopaths later on in life.

Feelings of abandonment, destruction, paranoia, depression, guilt and reparation are as old as the psyche itself—according to Melanie Klein (1992; 1993). These complicated feelings repeat throughout life, especially when unconscious infantile memories of abandonment and /or destruction get stirred. Thus, Camus' complex emotions concerning both his mother and father might be interestingly theorized through a Kleinian theoretical lens. Throughout his work readers see hints of anguish over abandonment issues, depression, guilt, reparation. Camus' becomes increasingly concerned with destruction through violence. Camus' was an advocate of non-violence, especially in the context of the unrelenting bloodshed during the French-Algerian War.

During the covid crisis, many patients in the hospital and their families have exhibited the very feelings that Klein describes above. Families of covid patients tend to express emotions of abandonment, paranoia, depression and survivor's guilt. Those who cannot tolerate uncomfortable emotions upon the death of a loved one often resort to violence. As I sat in a consult room with a family and the attending physician who explained the dire situation at hand as their loved one was dying from covid, one of the family members looked as if he was about to punch me in the stomach. I came to find out that his father—who was dying of covid—was a minister. The son must have made some kind of connection between his father and me—the chaplain—and wanted to punch me. This could have been an act of negative transference. Ten minutes later, it was reported that the son left the consult room, went outside the hospital into the parking lot and began punching the wall. This seems an irrational response to death and dying, but it is common. Many men—who have been taught not to cry—are enraged when a family member dies. Rage is the only emotion available to them. Rage is the most primary emotion we have and usually is the first one expressed for those who have been taught that to display emotion is not masculine. Perhaps after some time, anguish and depression set in.

Camus loved his mother, in fact he anguished over her silences and lack of emotion, her indifference. Interestingly, the sea—which could be considered a symbol of indifference—is a repeated metaphor for Camus throughout his work. In French, the words sea and mother share linguistic similarities (*la mer*= the sea; *la mere*=the mother).

Camus grew up in a sea of illiteracy as is reflected in his fictive or veiled autobiography "where there were no newspapers, nor, until Jacques brought them in, any books, no radio either, where there were only objects of immediate utility" (Camus, 1995 p. 202). Becoming a writer and philosopher could have been a response to his childhood where there little intellectual activity occurred. To grow up in a home without books or newspapers might lead to curiosity about things. Books open worlds. Camus—in a move of psychological reversal—became exactly what his mother was not, a voracious reader and writer.

As Camus progressed at the Lycee, "the silence grew between him and his family" (p. 203). Interestingly, Paul Viallaneix (1977), comments that

> Camus's work, more than any other, is born of silence. As far as he could reach back into his memories, indeed, he would run up against the absence or the impotence of language. He was unable to recall anything his father said. He was raised by a mother condemned to be mute by who knows what inhibition of the voice. He suffered from the inadequacy of her conversation. (p. 30)

This deafening silence—of a father killed in WWI when Camus was an infant and a mother who rarely spoke—would become part of Camus' philosophical views. A concept important to Camus is the absurd. In *The Myth of Sisyphus,* Camus (1955/1983) states: "The absurd is born of this confrontation between the human need and the unreasonable silence of the world" (p. 28). The silent world of Camus' childhood became etched in the text of his oeuvre; the absurd was the silent world impressed upon Camus' childhood and then unconsciously, or consciously expressed throughout his writings. It is interesting to note that Camus' psychic wounds as a child who grew up in a silent and indifferent world would serve him well later in life as he turned to writing. We have seen this pattern with others in this book who have also suffered traumatic childhoods who later became writers, namely, Louise DeSalvo and Derrick Jensen. DeSalvo often commented that writing was a way to heal.

So too for this book, writing is a way of healing from all of the trauma I have witnessed as a hospital chaplain, especially during the covid pandemic. I often ask myself, what do I do with all of this emotion? How do I take this emotion in without being destroyed emotionally. The very act of writing this book is an act not only of responsibility—to archive this horrific pandemic—but it is also an act of healing, or at least the attempt to heal from all that I have seen. I have often remarked elsewhere that I have seen things nobody should ever see. Walking outside of the hospital walls the world does seem a silent and indifferent place.

Other chaplains have said similar things to me: how do I even talk to people in the world outside of here, outside of the hospital walls? There seems a chasm between the hospital walls and the outside world. There is no form of education that might glue those worlds together, because there isn't any glue to begin with. We use theoretical frameworks in scholarship to glue ideas together but sometimes those frameworks fall apart as we simply cannot make our way through the world without the traces of the covid word lingering in our psyches.

An entire world seemed silent and indifferent—to Camus—in the face of inhumanity and tragedy. However, just as Camus made his way— accepting his mother's silence and indifference—he also used these psychic wounds in the service of writing. Camus became one of the greatest novelists and philosophers of his generation. Meursault –in *The Stranger*—states that he is finally able to "[lay his heart] open to the benign indifference of the universe" (cited in Viallaneix, 1977, p. 98). And yet "Meursault wavers between yes and no until his death" (cited in Viallaneix, 1977, p. 98). The "yes and no" might signify *mourning*— a *yes*, which for Freud (1916) means working through; and a *no*—in the form of *melancholia*—which for Freud (1917) means an inability to work through (psychic problems).

Camus (1977) writes in a short essay: "He had a mother. Sometimes she would be asked a question: 'What are you thinking about?'- 'Nothing', she would answer.—And it was very true" (p. 30).

Perhaps it was "nothing" this no-response, this lack of words which, ironically, gave Camus the gift of language and writing. Camus (1955/1983,) in *The Myth of* Sisyphus, again, writes about thinking about nothing:

> In certain situations, replying "nothing" when asked what one is thinking about may be a pretense.... But if the reply is sincere, if it symbolizes that odd state of soul in which the void becomes eloquent, in which the chain of daily gestures is broken... it is as it were the first sign of absurdity. (p. 12)

Psychoanalyst Christopher Bollas (1986) recalls Paula Heimann—who asked a rhetorical question that is relevant to Camus' words: "To whom is this person speaking?" (cited in Bollas, 1986, p. 1). Was Camus speaking to the one who could not be addressed, as Derrida (1987) might put it? Derrida (1987) writes in *The Post Card*

> Who is writing? To whom? And to send, to destine, to dispatch what? To what address? Without any desire or surprise, and thereby to grab attention by means of obscurity. (p. 5)

Camus' writings are akin to Derrida's post card that is never received, or the post card that is never understood. Like the person who writes a post card, Camus' writing is terse, his sentences tight. As if writing on a post card, there is no room for flowery language. The person writing the post card must get to the point, waste no words. Camus never wasted a word, not one. Exquisite. A style so terse, sparse; it is crystal clear like the crystal-clear blue sea—reflecting the Mediterranean of his childhood.

Camus' writings reflect an intense passion for living. But his passion for living was tempered by memories of growing up in poverty during war. Again, the yes and the no. Camus (1977) states:

> We are in life. It strikes us, mutilates us, spits in our face. It also illuminates us with crazy and sudden happiness that makes us participants. It is short. That is enough. Still, make no mistake: there is pain. Impossible to evade. Perhaps, deep within ourselves, life's essential lot. (p. 210)

This back and forth movement in his thought—life's horrors, life's happiness—to lose things and to find things, to roll the rock up the hill, to have it smash us on the way down only to start over again—this is Sisyphus' tragic fate. Camus identified psychologically with Sisyphus. And yet Camus did not become a nihilist. Likewise, In *The Rebel: An Essay on Man in Revolt* Camus (1956/1991), asserts: "What is a rebel? A man who says no, but whose refusal does not imply a renunciation. He is also a man who says yes, from the moment he makes his first gesture of rebellion" (p. 13). A yes and a no. The continual dialectic. Camus, in fact, wrote a piece titled "Between yes and no" (cited in Bree, 1972. P. 57). Germaine Bree (1972) states that

> Camus's childhood eluded him. Again and again he grappled with it. Around his twentieth year he seems to have thought of fictionalizing it in a novel, a project he abandoned, but to the substance of which he had returned at the time of his death. *La Mort heureuse* is a novel of initiation into manhood. (p. 57)

It is interesting to note that Camus wanted to write his memoir, which later became *The First Man* (*La Mort Heureuse*), when he was only twenty years old. Then he dropped the idea for decades. Why would one want to write a memoir while one is still so young? And then, why would one drop the idea altogether for decades? Is it because his childhood "eluded" him, as Bree (1972, p. 57) suggests?

On some level, everyone's' childhood "elude[s]" them. But on another level, there are some things about childhood that can be made sense of—even if one's childhood is awful. Who knows what Camus understood about his childhood—perhaps it "eluded" him or perhaps not. It is impossible to know. One thing is clear: Camus put his childhood memories to psychological use. D.W. Winnicott (1970) often asked to what use does one put psychological problems? Andre Green (1993) suggests that creativity springs from trauma:

> The compromised unity of the ego which has a hole in it from now on, realizes itself either on the level of fantasy, which gives open expression to artistic creation, or on the level of knowledge, which is at the origin of highly productive intellectualization. It is evident that one is witnessing an attempt to master the traumatic situation. (p. 153)

Does one engage in the very act of writing about living through a pandemic—such as the covid crisis—in order to "master the traumatic situation"? I know I cannot "master" this "traumatic situation" but the writing about it and writing through it give me a way to organize a disorganized world, a world in utter disarray. Writing is a way to organize—or order—one's chaotic thoughts. Even if this is a futile attempt to make sense of what cannot be made sense of, still it is an ethical responsibility to archive the traces of this pandemic for future generations. And perhaps that is why writers like Camus, DeSalvo and Jensen became writers; partly to organize their worlds, to make sense of chaos and to leave behind an archive for others. Of course I cannot speak for others, but I will say that those who have lived through trauma—whether it stems from horrific childhoods or becoming unglued from working on covid wards—writing things out is a way of releasing negative transference.

Curiously, Bree (1972) claims that Camus hid in his writing. Bree states "Camus found it difficult to project himself directly into his writing. This led him, on occasion, to hide deeply personal reactions under a cloak of impersonal rhetoric" (p. 57). Did Camus consciously work at absenting himself from his writing? Camus states: "Gide has strived too much for distance from Gide. This is the aspect of Gide I immediately understood. But isn't this because I am looking for a way to become distant from myself?" (in Viallaneix, 1977, pp. 179-180). Did Camus wish to become "distant" from himself to distance himself from his painful childhood? Or, did Camus—perhaps unconsciously—want to mirror his distant mother?

Camus (1955/1983) claims that *the* problem for a philosopher is suicide. In *The Myth of Sisyphus*—Camus states: "There is but one truly serious philosophical problem, and that is suicide" (p. 3). Yes, Camus—himself—might have had many reasons to die by suicide. His childhood seemed a hopeless nothingness, dead. His mother was emotionally dead to him. Many children who grow up with emotionally absent mothers do not do so well in adult life. They either resort to repeating that deadness in some way, or wish that they were literally dead. Andre Green (1993) claims that "there is no end to the dead mother's dying… It is a hurt on the edge of a wound" (p. 153). That "hurt on the edge of a wound" seemed to haunt Camus throughout his life. Death, murder and suicide—wounded subjects—are important themes for Camus. But perhaps these topics were of importance to Camus—not for literal reasons—but as metaphors of limit experiences. The absurd, Camus' major concept, signifies limit experiences.

Camus' *The Plague* and Archiving the Covid Pandemic

In *The Plague* (1947), Camus begins with a seemingly innocuous event. "When leaving his surgery on the morning of April 16, Dr. Bernard Rieux felt something soft under his foot. It was a dead rat lying in the middle of the landing" (p. 7). The dead rat—a nuisance—signifies the beginning of a plague that kills nearly everyone in the town of Oran. The narrator say that Oran "strikes" one in its "ordinariness" (p. 3). It is in the ordinary that life and death happen—Camus suggests. Life and death, ironically, are hardly ordinary—however. Living as if one is dead is what makes life and death seem ordinary.

Jean Tarrou, who calls himself "the writer," in Camus' (1947) *The Plague,* sees his task as a kind of archivist, or historian who "had a habit of observing events and people through the wrong lens of the telescope" (p. 22). This "chronicler" (p. 22) records "seeming-trivial details" (p. 22). Tarrou "set himself to recording the history of what the normal historian passes over" (p. 22). I identify with Tarrou as I too am attempting to "chronicle" events of the covid pandemic that the "normal historian" will ignore. Most historians do not use first-person (witness) accounts, especially if the person writing the account is traumatized. Those who have suffered through traumatic events—most historians would say—cannot be trusted because their memories are not reliable. But who would know more about the traumatic even than the one who lived through it? Historians put under erasure the voices of those who need to be heard the most. This book is not about getting the story right; this book is not about being a reliable narrator. This book is about archiving a trauma as it is unfolding so as to capture—in the present—what is happening. After the covid crisis is over—and we hope that one day it will be—these memories will fade. Fading memories are lost memories. Archiving history as it unfolds is a difficult task, indeed. One might ask if the present is history at all? When does history become history? For me, history begins the moment that the very moment passes in time. The clock ticking is history.

Derrida (1996) remarks that the archive is reflective of the flow of time, both backwards—as a form of memory work—and forward, as a responsibility to the future, to future generations. Derrida (1996) declares:

> And the word and the notion of the archive seem at first, admittedly, to point toward the past, to refer the signs of consigned memory, to recall faithfulness to tradition.... As much as and more than a thing of the past, the archive should call into question the coming of the future. (pp. 33-34)

The archivist—who lives in the present, in the now—also lives in the past, through archival work—but must anticipate the responsibility to the future as those who will live in the future will look back to the past as the archivist saw it, as the archivist represented the past. This movement of archivization is hardly static, it is, rather, again, circular. Is this not the movement of Pinar's (2006) notion of *Currere*? Currere is the autobiographical and psychic movement between one's past, one's present and one's future. But not only that, *currere*—reflects cultural and social movement—a historicity, if you will. The self does not live in a vacuum, but in a socio-political world that is always already historical.

The way in which Derrida (1996) conceptualizes the archive is in contradistinction to the Hegelian (1977) philosophy of history in *Phenomenology of Spirit* whereby events—in continual contradiction—eventually press toward the future of the Spirit or the Idea. Hegel's is an Enlightenment model of history whereby progress looks to the future as Spirit comes to know itself through self-consciousness. Hegel's (1977) is a progress narrative, even though it is dialectical. Derrida (1994), much Foucault (1994), stresses the necessity of thinking things historically. Foucault importantly points out that the way that history gets archived is completely ambiguous. Memoirists—who look back upon their lives—as well as historians pick and choose what is to be included and what is excluded from the historical narrative. These decisions of what to include or exclude are subjective. History is not linear either. The way that history unfolds is quite complicated and beyond the scope of this book. The point I am attempting to drive home is that archiving a traumatic event—like the pandemic—as it unfolds, is completely arbitrary. What gets excluded from the archive is perhaps unconscious material that is not yet able to be digested psychically.

Walter Benjamin's (1999) in *Arcades Project* focused on objects from mundane experiences; he magnified the mundane, he let the objects speak as it were. Benjamin's objects tell a kind of story. Street lamps, dolls, arcades, gas lanterns and so forth are a kind of archive-of-objects which reflect a time in history that is no more. His love affair with Paris is archived through the Parisian objects he found on the street. Perhaps the object of this book is the virus—an invisible object, a thing that invades the body. A microscopic object that kills. The question is: for how long? How many more years do we have to endure the horrors of the object that kills? The virus that has stolen so many lives.

Camus' (1947) *The Plague* deals with issues like time, which has everything to do with historicity and archivization. During the plague—the sense of time changed, Camus' narrator tells us. Everyone knew that they could die next. The rats died in droves, and then people began dying in droves. Waiting to be the next victim of plague is akin to Dante's *Inferno*. The famous opening lines in Dante's prose-poem are fitting: All ye who enter here lose hope. The loss of hope, continual death, no end in sight: that is the experience of living through a plague. Time—in that Inferno, in that Plague is no longer experienced as progressing, or moving at all. Time stops. The virus stops time and yet years pass. Time moves slowly, more people succumb to the virus. Time moves backwards as we attempt to capture the stories of the pandemic. The narrator of Camus' story states:

> Without memories, without hope, they lived for the moment only. Indeed, the here and now had come to mean everything for them.... nothing was left for us but a series of present moments. (p. 165)

Time drags during a pandemic, during our pandemic, covid 19. Time drags and feels as if it has come to a standstill. Especially, if one gets sick from covid. The days turn into more days, the days turn into months, everything is the same every day because being sick stops time. One day is like the next, one night is the same as the day. This is a strange phenomenon when one gets ill. Time has become stagnant, without flow.

What Camus' narrator describes as time experienced as "a series of present moments" (p. 165) is not unlike the way ancient Greek philosopher Parmenides wrote about time. He states: "being has no coming-into-being and no destruction, for it is whole of limb, without motion, and without end. And it never was, nor will be, because it is now, a whole all together, one, continuous [reality]" (in Kaufman, 1968, p. 20). Parmenides is one of the few ancient Greek philosophers who thought that time was still, motionless, without movement. This is a difficult idea with which to grapple. Although Parmenides' ideas have been thought misguided, they are good metaphors for experiencing illness. When getting sick from covid—as I did twice—I was stuck, and isolated, in the same room for months and months, without being able to do much. Brain fog and exhaustion are what covid brings and time is experienced as Parmenides writes about it.

The Physician and the Priest

The roles of both physician and priest are similar: they are healers. The physician heals the body; the priest heals the soul. However, there is, historically, a tension and even a resentment between the physician and priest, as I mentioned in an earlier chapter in this book. Science and religion can move in counter-directions. The religious seek miracles; scientists seek knowledge. Belief and reason do not always make good bedfellows.

Camus—throughout his work—depict scientists as heroes, while religious figures are evil; they are portrayed as ignorant and cruel. Two major characters in *The Plague* bear this out. Dr. Bernard Rieux—the healer of bodies—does the hard work of taking care of patients in a no-win situation, but he keeps doing his job no matter. He is persistent, deliberate, thoughtful. Dr. Rieux is the hero. Contrarily, the priest, Father Paneloux is ignorant, irrational, and cruel. Father Paneloux's character is similar to the chaplain in Camus' (1946/1989) *The Stranger*. He, too, acted out of ignorance and cruelty.

Raymond Rambert—the journalist—accuses Dr. Rieux of living in a world of "abstractions" (p. 78). Rambert says, "No... you can't understand. You're using the language of reason, not of the heart; you live in a world of abstractions" (p. 78). It is ironic that the one who engages with the dying, is accused of living in a world of abstractions. What can be more human than tending to the dying? An attending physician, *tends* to the dying. However, medical science is based on abstractions and concepts, but these abstractions and concepts are put to work in the tending to patients. Physicians straddle two worlds: the abstractions of the science of medicine, and taking care of human beings.

To take care and tend to the sick is to tend to human beings. Medicine is not simply the art of being compassionate; it is also the art of knowing—through medical science—how to put abstractions to work. Dr. Rieux—level-headed, rational and knowing cares for his patients until the end of the plague.

Camus certainly was the least abstract philosopher of his generation. However, Camus' work is not easy to understand, either. I find some of his texts quite obscure, in fact. Camus' literary fiction is not easy to decipher. Questioning the inhumane troubled Camus the most. Camus was, indeed, a humanist.

The narrator of Camus' (1947) *The Plague* tells us that Dr. Rieux "was conscious of a bleak indifference steadily gaining on him" (p. 83). Here again the notion of indifference emerges. Indifference—as a philosophical stance, or even a way of being-in-the-world—has a long tradition in the history of philosophy. One can trace the notion of indifference—as a quality to be admired, rather than something to be shunned—back to the Stoics, the Skeptics and the Cynics. Epictetus, for example, stated

> Withdraw, therefore, your aversion from all matters that are not under our control, and transfer it to what is unnatural among those which are under our control. But for the time being remove utterly your desire; for if you desire some one of the things that are not under our control you are bound to be unfortunate. (1968, p. 478)

Walter Kaufman (1968) comments that "Looking back on the development of Greek philosophy from the pre-Socratics to the Stoics, the Epicureans, and the Skeptics, one is struck by the overwhelming concern of the later schools with peace of mind" (p. 451). Michel Foucault (2012) was particularly drawn to the Cynics—in his late lectures—as he remarked that Diogenes—the Cynic—felt that dogs lived the best kind of life, for they live a life of indifference. In fact, the word Cynic, as Kaufman (1968) points out, means "doglike" in Greek (p. 449). Dogs are indifferent to praise or blame, and therefore, they are free from dread and angst, worry and so forth. Whether these claims are true or not is a question, perhaps, for another day.

At any rate, all of these schools of ancient philosophy might be traced back to Socrates, especially in Plato's (2008) *Apology*. Socrates is put on trial and sentenced to death for corrupting the youth; he calmly states that although the charges brought against him are false, he willingly goes to his death because he knows that he spoke truth to power and he was willing to die for the truth. Further, for Socartes, death means little because he argues that death is either like sleep or it is another realm where philosophical conversations—in an afterlife—can be carried on with philosophers who have died. After death, that is, the philosophical conversations will continue with the dead. Socrates' attitude toward death is one of stoic acceptance; Socrates was not afraid of death.

Indifference towards death—a belief held by the Stoics, Cynics, Skeptics and Socrates—was probably not unfamiliar to Camus. However, I do not know whether these various schools of philosophical indifference and/or Socrates influenced Camus' writings.

It is interesting to note that the life of indifference can be traced to the monastic Fathers and Mothers of the Desert in ancient Christian culture about whom I wrote in an earlier chapter in this book. However, I do not think Camus had much truck with religion or Christianity; the religious figures in his novels are painted in a negative light, as I said earlier.

The archivization of the past must be broad and inclusive. I have argued in this chapter that it is important not to ignore biographies and autobiographies when engaging in archiving history. This, however, is still a contentious issue with professional philosophers, who by and large, do not see the point of biography. Many professional philosophers remain formalists and feel that the only thing that really matters is the text, not the context in which the text had been written. And here, I think professional philosophers—those who feel this way—are mistaken. Derrida (1996) speaks to these issues:

> And if we still lack a viable, unified, given concept of the archive, it is undoubtedly not a purely conceptual, theoretical, espistemological insufficiency on the level of multiple and specific disciplines; it is perhaps not for lack of sufficient elucidation in certain circumscribed domains: archeology, documentography, bibliography, philology, historiography. (p. 34)

I note two important biographies of Derrida here. Benoit Peeters' (2013) *Derrida: A Biography* and Peter Salmon's (2020) work *An Event, Perhaps: A Biography of Jacques Derrida*. Biographies of philosophers have become a more accepted genre, say, within the last decade. But whether professional philosophers think that they have much relevance against the actual work of philosophy—the texts at hand—is another question altogether. Biographies are forms of archivization. So too are memoirs and autobiographies. Even fictionalized autobiographies—like Camus' (1995) *The First Man*—tell us something about the person (the who) that writes the text (the what)—as Derrida (2003) put it. It is interesting that Freud was skeptical of biographies because he understood that a biography is a social construction and is shot through with mimesis and transference. Still, biography—given that it is speculation, a social construction and is intricately related—in many ways—to the biographer and her own life history—it is still an important form of archivization.

Had I not studied Camus' biographic situation, perhaps my reading of him would be more naïve. The context of a person's life history does matter when studying their writings. Context tells us something about the text-at-hand. However, professional philosophers—for the most part—still feel that biography is beside the point, it does not mean much against the work of doing philosophy. I beg to differ with professional philosophers on this point.

Camus' Father Paneloux

Camus' most virulent critiques in his literary fiction are directed at the religious. In *The Plague*, Camus' ire against the religious is directed against the priest, Father Paneloux. The narrator of *The Plague* states "But where some saw abstractions others saw the truth" (p. 84). Here, the narrator is actually critiquing those who think they know the truth with a capital T. This kind of truth, is the truth of absolutism about which Camus was highly critical. The sadistic priest Father Paneloux, embraced an absolutist stance on the truth. This was something Camus abhorred.

Truth with a capital T, absolutist truth is in the service of destructive forms of power. Nietzsche's (2017) will to power—when aligned with the will to truth—leads to fascism. Robert Musil (1996)—in his novel *The Man without Qualities*—speaks to Nietzsche's concern. Musil, an Austrian novelist—who lived in the early 20th century—anticipated the rise of Fascism in Europe, especially in his home country of Austria. Musil's novel was banned—according to Burton Pike (1996)—in both Austria and Germany during the Third Reich. Musil's thesis is that identity-politics (a kind of will to power in collision with the will to truth) leads to nationalism, fascism, and worse. That is, being self-certain and absolutistic about one's identity and one's nationality leads to practices of Othering, destruction and war. Musil claims—in *The Man Without Qualities*—that it is better to be uncertain of oneself (i.e. to be a man without qualities), than to be absolutistic—about anything, identity, truth, nationality and so forth.

Father Paneloux in Camus' *The Plague* represents the antithesis of Musil's man without qualities, for Paneloux represents a person blinded by his own collision with the will to truth and the will to power. Father Paneloux's dogmatic religious beliefs lead to ignorance and cruelty. Religious dogma was partly to blame, too, for the rise of Nazism. Both Catholic and Protestant Churches hung Swastikas from their windows. Christian anti-Semitism and ethnic anti-Semitism was enmeshed with Hitler's Final Solution. Even the Confessing Church—the church to which Dietrich Bonhoeffer belonged— was mostly sympathetic to Hitler's regime. The myth of the Confessing Church had been—-for decades—that it was one of the few churches that led a resistance movement against Hitler. But this myth has recently been debunked. Although Bonhoeffer was involved in the foiled plot to kill Hitler, and although he was a member of the Confessing Church, most members of that church were anti-Semitic and actually sympathetic to Hitler's Final Solution. Even the Pope, as historian Susan Zuccotti (2002) points out—was not an innocent bystander; in fact, he was a collaborator.

Camus' Father Paneloux's diatribes are remarkably similar to the philosophical tracts of Liebniz (2020). Leibnix claimed that everything that happened in the world was God's will; nothing happened because of chance. Paneloux rants—in essence—that the Plague was God's will and all "evildoers" deserve to die.

> The just man need have no fear, but the evildoer has good cause to tremble. For plague is the flail of God and the world his threshing-floor. (p. 87)

Paneloux rants that those who succumb to the plague deserve it: they deserve God's wrath because they are "evildoer[s]." Many evangelical preachers during the AIDS epidemic blamed gay men for contracting AIDS and said that Gay men deserved to die because they were abominations. The notorious Father Coughlin (on a radio show listened to by millions of Americans) in the United States, railed against the Jews during the 1930s and 1940s—during the Holocaust and blamed the Jews for their own demise because they were evil. More recently, Nation of Islam leader The "Honorable" Reverend Farrakhan—as his followers call him, has ranted—in public forums—that Jews are agents of Satan. Farrakhan was banned from Facebook for engaging in such outrageous anti-Semitic rants.

Like Camus, Bertrand Russell (1957) exclaims that

> Christian ideology and dogma is Only a rationalization of sadism.... I would invite any Christian to accompany me to the children's ward of a hospital, to watch the suffering that is there being endured, and then to persist in the assertion that those children are so morally abandoned as to deserve what they are suffering. (p. 30)

Russell's anger is wholly justified and still relevant against the backdrop of the covid pandemic. In the third year of this horror, medical professionals report that many children are being admitted to ICUs; some are on ventilators, some are even dying from covid. Bertrand Russell (1957) points out, God must be "sadistic" (p. 30), to allow for the suffering and death of children. The problem of evil—a discipline called theodicy— critiques and puts into question religious dogma that blames victims for their own demise (because they are evil or abominations) during pandemics, plagues and other atrocities.

Camus' Father Paneloux proclaims: "Calamity has come on you, my brethren, and, my brethren, you deserved it." (pp. 86-87). Camus has no truck with the abuses of religion. Camus paints Father Paneloux in the worst possible light in *The Plague;* indeed, Father Paneloux is—himself—the most evil character in Camus' novel.

The Plague and Authoritarianism

Camus' *The Plague* is also interpreted as a metaphor for the rise of authoritarianism. Hannah Arendt (1979) wrote one of the most important works on authoritarianism in the 20th century, in *The Origins of Totalitarianism.* When historians discuss Hitler's rise to power, they tell us that many thought he would just go away. Many European intellectuals felt this too. But Arendt warned her intellectual colleagues that they might pay more attention to politics in their work. Philosophy and psychoanalysis for that matter, were hardly political during the 1930s. Even Freud and Adorno thought that Hitler would just go away. But some, like Walter Benjamin, did not think that; nor did Arendt. There is an expression in Germany that Hitler's his reign of terror happened as if people were asleep. Untoward events seem to happen slowly—like the emergence of the rats in Camus' *The Plague.* When the first rat is stepped on and squashed—in Camus' novel by Dr. Rieux, he did not pay much attention. But then more and more rats appeared dead, in garbage cans, on the streets, everywhere. Fascism happens one rat at a time, it seems. But before you know it, thousands of dead rats appear everywhere. Laws are passed, one by one, ghettos are built, concentration camps are built, trains begin transporting people to extermination camps. Authoritarianism is a plague: and it is always already closer to us—in time- than we might think. Plagues return, pandemics have always been with us. They come back, albeit in different forms: plagues and pandemics are akin to the return of the repressed, as Freud would put it. Authoritarianism, too, comes back: it, too, is the return of the repressed. The collision of covid-19 and the authoritarian regime of former President Trump escalated the death-by-numbers of covid victims during the first year of the pandemic, because nothing was done, at first. Over 600 thousand people died within a little over one year. Three years into the pandemic and the numbers in the United States are veering toward one million deaths.

The Stranger

Like Camus' (1947) *The Plague*, *The Stranger* (1946/1989) begins in the most seemingly ordinary way. Meursault receives a telegram that his mother had just died. A telegram is like a post card. It is a seemingly innocuous form of communication. And yet... the news of Mersault's mother's death, is hardly ordinary or innocuous. Meursault—strangely—however, thinks that his mother's death is the most ordinary of events.

> Maman died today. Or yesterday maybe, I don't know. I got a telegram from home: "Mother deceased. Funeral tomorrow. Faithfully yours." That doesn't mean anything. Maybe it was yesterday. (Camus, 1946/1989 p. 3)

Meursault is indifferent to the fact that *"maman"* was dead. He does not know exactly when she died and does not seem to care; nor does her death or the funeral "mean anything." At the funeral, Meursault "hadn't cried once" (p. 89). Similarly, Camus' (1977), about his own mother? proclaims: "There! She's dead. Isn't she? I won't see her anymore. I love her. She dies.... But she is dead. Yesterday she moved" (p. 200). Camus focuses on a mother who is dead.

The indifference and distance Camus creates between the narrator and his mother's death emerges in both *The Stranger* and *The Presence of the Dead* (1977). Can one love the dead? Can one love the (psychically) dead? Being alive and yet dead (physically) is confusing—especially for a child. Meursault—in *The Stranger*—is put on trial and convicted—not for murdering a man—but—absurdly—for *not* crying at his mother's funeral. Meursault is indifferent. Killing a man did not seem to mean much to him either. The man's death simply annoyed him—absurdly—because Mersault got overheated from the sun.

The ancient Greek cynic Diogenes—with whom Foucault (2012) identified—stated to Alexander the Great, "get out of my sunlight" (cited in Kaufman, 1968, p. 450). One does not say such things to Alexander the Great. What an absurd thing to say! But Diogenes was indifferent people's opinions of him; he proclaimed that he was like a dog, because a dog is indifferent to what anyone thinks.

In Camus' *The Stranger*, Mersault kills a man on the beach (who seems to be an abstraction, rather than a human). We come to find out that Mersault shot and killed an *Arab* man on the beach. Meursault was dead serious—when in court—he stated that it was the sun that made him pull the trigger because he was simply overheated and felt annoyed. Being annoyed does not seem a rational defense for murder. And this is what makes Camus' novel so strange.

As was mentioned earlier, it seems that Camus' philosophical position on indifference had much to do with the deep love and admiration of his mother who was, indeed, indifferent to the world. Camus' drew upon his relationship with his mother—especially in his childhood—for his writings.

Camus had an uncanny knack for cutting through things. He asked philosophical questions of relevance; he pondered questions of his time; he was a man of his time. For Camus, philosophical questions born of logic mattered little in a world of irrationality, absurdity and mindlessness, and meaninglessness. This—Camus—suggested throughout his writings, is an absurd world. In this sense, Camus had things in common with Franz Kafka—who thought that the world—in all its ridiculous bureaucracy—was absurd. But Camus, unlike Kafka, was not concerned with the problems of bureaucracy but the indifference of the world.

Camus' Self-Education

Olivier Todd (2000) states Louis Germain saw talent in Camus when he was attending primary school. It was Germain who encouraged Camus in his studies. Poverty, however, got in the way. Camus' mother—who was not indifferent to Camus' education—approached Germain about securing a scholarship for her son's high school education. However, the fierce matriarch of the house, Camus' grandmother

> was against scholarships for Albert, feeling that he should work for his living the way Lucien [Camus's brother] did. But with Catherine Helen's [Camus' mother] encouragement, Germaine explained about the boy's skill in reading, writing, and the spoken word, and that the scholarship would pay for a high-school diploma, after which Albert could get a better job. (Todd, 2000, p. 1)

When a child from a working-class family (like Camus) advances through education it is not uncommon—if I may generalize for a moment—for family members to feel resentment. Perhaps his grandmother felt resentment because her grandson would advance into the world of the learned. Camus had no great love for his grandmother. Germaine Bree (1974) comments that

> Beyond the crude realities of working-class life... he [Camus] perceived another reality, incarnated in his mother... I was the way of life of tenacious men and women, anonymous and stoical, working in poverty for their bare subsistence.

Cruelty and suffering for them were things to be endured. Camus himself, at seventeen, would endure alone and in silence, the physical reality of the tuberculosis gnawing at his lungs. (p. 63)

Camus knew sickness. Like Marcel Proust—who also suffered from tuberculosis—both became introspective writers. One must wonder what the connection might be between sickness and writing. Perhaps that link (between sickness and writing) is the development of a keen sense of turning inward. When one is ill, time is all you have. Time, in fact, slows down. Illness turns one to the world within. Of course, not all people who succumb to illness become writers; but there are many writers who have succumbed to illness, Proust being one. Camus being another. Tuberculosis—about which Thomas Mann (1996) wrote in his novel *Magic Mountain*—was another European pandemic in the late 19th century. The great Indian mathematician Ramanujan—who cracked the code of partition theory and broke ground for mathematical formulas which later became a foundational for the study of black holes—succumbed both to tuberculosis and hepatic amebiasis that killed him. Walter Benjamin suffered from heart trouble, which made his attempt to escape the Nazis impossible; however it was not heart trouble that killed him, he died by suicide. Freud suffered from cancer of the jaw and in stated that he could not work without being in some kind of pain.

Like many of these other intellectuals who succumbed to illness—and yet persisted to become writers, philosophers, mathematicians, founders of intellectual movements like psychoanalysis and so forth, despite Camus' struggles with tuberculosis he persisted and became a writer and philosopher. Yet, unlike these other intellectuals, Camus felt that he was self-educated, a kind of organic intellectual; in fact, like a character in Greek myth, he felt that he birthed himself. Hence the title of his fictional memoir, *The First Man*. Bree (1974) states: "There were no mirrors or books in Albert Camus's home" (p. 62). Camus (1995) states: " What has helped me bear an adverse fate will perhaps help me accept an overly favorable outcome—and what has most sustained me was the great vision, the very great vision I have of art" (p. 320).

Critiques of Camus

Postcolonial scholars are highly critical of Camus. During the French-Algerian war and before, he intimated that Arab-Algerians could not sustain an independent Algeria. Postcolonial scholars point out that for Camus, liberty, equality, fraternity was a slogan meant for the French, not for Arab-Algerians. Many postcolonial scholars, therefore, call Camus out for his racism and his islamophobia. Camus' stand on Algerian independence has come back to haunt him. Ena Vulor (2000) states:

> Camus's narratives continue to be read today within a purely French literary tradition, as parables of the human condition. The choice of an Algerian setting appears almost incidental to the pressing issues of man's alienated condition. (xxiv-xxv)

Camus writes about the human condition-writ large—he called himself a humanist. Some intellectuals say that Camus was the conscience of his generation. But it is important to contextualize his work against the French-Algerian war and the long-standing anti-Arab sentiment that many French have had against native Algerians since at least the French colonization of Algeria. Vulor (2000) points out that

> During his last years, as he increasingly withdrew from direct political action, he sought refuge in a strongly moralistic humanism. His refusal to support the Algerian rebels during the French-Algerian war received bitter reproaches from left-wing politicians. (p. xix)

Postcolonial scholars—especially—consider Camus to be little more than a hypocrite. Freedom for the French; colonization for the Arab. European humanism—as it is traditionally conceived—is, indeed, racist, classist and sexist. Even worse, humanism can be construed as "monstrous." Sartre in 1961—in the preface to Frantz Fanon's (1963) *Wretched of the Earth*—said of humanism that it created "monsters" (p. 26). Sartre sums it up here:

> Is Europe any different? And that super-European monstrosity, North America? Chatter, chatter: liberty, equality, fraternity, love, honour, patriotism... All of this did not prevent us from making anti-racial speeches about dirty niggers, dirty Jews and dirty Arabs.... there is nothing more consistent than a racist humanism since Europe has only been able to become a man through creating slaves and monsters. (pp. 25-26)

This pointed critique of humanism is applicable to the tradition of Western philosophy as well. Postcolonial scholarship has upended the Western philosophical tradition, and rightly so. Western philosophy is highly problematic as it is a canon of mostly White European males, who were also racist, sexist, homophobic, islamaphobic and anti-Semitic.

Some postcolonial scholars have noted that throughout Camus' novels, Arabs are faceless. The facelessness of Arab characters is associated with Camus' racism and islamophobia. Richard Keller (2007) points out that "Emily Apter's work on Camus, for example, highlights the "nullification of Arab Characters in his works: Algerian Arabs are either absent or appear only as underdeveloped set decoration" (p. 8). Likewise, in much non-Jewish German fiction after the Holocaust Jews are faceless or they are mentioned in passing. Facelessness signifies erasure, racism, anti-Semitism or worse (Morris, 2001). For example, it is notable that in the novels of Gunter Grass (1959)—especially the *Tin Drum*—Jews are but background material and are faceless.

It has been noted in the popular press that Camus is not taught in Algerian schools because he is considered the face of French colonization.

For a variety of reasons—including colonialism—Craig DeLancey (2019) in, *Quillette*, remarks that "[f]or the most of his life... Camus was deeply unfashionable among France's leading intellectuals. In many quarters he still is" (np). Patricia Lorcin (2014) in *The South Central Review* explains:

> Certainly the break with Sartre was instrumental in exacerbating the condemnation of Camus as a died-in-the-wool colonist. Camus' denunciation of revolution... and his condemnation of the excess of Stalinism set the stage. (p. 12)

"Camus' disavowal of revolution seemed as 'naïve' to Sartre" (cited in Delancey, 2019, np). While Sartre and de Beauvoir were blinded by Communism's promises, Camus, along with Richard Wright—the African American novelist—were cautious and, in many ways, anticipated the horrors of Stalin. It is a most interesting fact that today Russia or what is called the Russian Federation—wrote out of its constitution—that the driving ideology of Russia is communism anymore. Thus, the Russian Federation paints itself as a non-communist country. However, Putin—in many ways—acts like Stalin as he throws his critics in Gulag-like prisons never to be seen again; he quells dissent by imprisoning and even killing his opponents. It is no accident that those who Putin fears mysteriously fall out of windows, or die by poisoned tea. Is this not the way Stalin ran the Communist Soviet Union? Putin acts as if he were still a KGB agent. At any rate, Camus was right about the way in which communist ideologies got played out in state politics; Sartre and de Beauvoir got it wrong. It is important to draw a distinction between the writings of Marx (1976)—in particular his *Communist*

Manifesto—and the way in which communism played out in state politics and got twisted into something it was never meant to be—on a careful reading of the writings of Marx.

Academic philosophers—at least in the United States—have tended to shun Marx as well as Camus because neither fits into the accepted canon of philosophy. Professional philosophy has become increasingly narrow, uber-technical and elitist. Perhaps it is time to think otherwise. Although Camus' colonialism is in need of critique, I do not think he should be erased from the canon. Many European philosophers have been racist, sexist and anti-Semitic. However, erasing people from the canon presents yet another problem of exclusion. If we continue to exclude those we find fault with, soon there will be no one left. However, I am certainly not condoning reprehensible behavior, or racism sexism, islamophobic or anti-Semitism. These things must continually be roundly critiqued. But if texts that we inherit are worthwhile studying, if history is worthwhile studying, if the history of the archive of texts is worthwhile studying, we critique and then build from what we find useful in that which we have inherited. Marx (1976) critiqued Hegel, but he built his work in contradistinction to Hegel, and in fact, drew quite heavily from Hegel especially in his *1844 Manuscripts*, which would become the basis of all of his writings. And yes, there are disturbing passages in Marx as well; passages that demand critique. But can we not critique and build or veer away from what Marx teaches? The same could be said of Camus' writings. Some of his ideas we must critique, some we build upon, and some move beyond. Camus is still worth studying, despite his horrid real-world politics.

Camus was a problematic figure. There is no denying his colonial stance—among other things. But dismissing his work out of hand is not a good option. Today—because of the covid pandemic and the and rise of global authoritarianism(s)—Camus' work has become increasingly relevant to our current global catastrophe.

8

Michel Serres' Relevance for Unbearable Stories of the Covid Pandemic

Throughout Michel Serres' work, references to the clinamen appear. Some suggest that the term first emerged in the writings of Epicurus (who lived around 340 BCE); others suggest Lucretius (2007)—an ancient poet (who lived around 400 BCE)—brought into conversation a similar term called the swerve in *De Rerum Natura* or *The Nature of Things*. According to Richard Jenkyns (2007) *De Rerum Nartura* was interrupted—perhaps unfinished—because of the plague that occurred in Athens around 430 BCE. This is significant for our purposes because the clinamen (or the swerve) are uncannily relevant to the covid-19 pandemic we are currently living through.

It is interesting to note that Michel Serres (2001) mentions plagues—especially in his work on ancient physics and philosophy. Plagues have a relation to the concept of the clinamen because they occur by chance happenings. In Lucretius' (2007) *De Rerum Natura* what Epicurus called the clinamen is referred to as "the swerve" (2007, p. 42). Lucretius (2007) proclaims

> *They swerve a little.* [meaning atoms] Just enough of a serve for you to call it a change of course. Unless inclined to swerve, all things would fall right through the deep abyss like drops of rain. There would be no collisions, and no atom with a blow, and Nature thus could not have fashioned anything, full stop. (p. 42)

Lucretius, although not writing about a plague, suggests that nature—generally speaking—comes into being because of a sheer accident as atoms crash into one another—these become the building blocks the very stuff of life. Life, in other words, is not divinely ordained; there is no prime mover who creates the universe. The universe is created by chance.

Atoms "swerve a little, but only by the smallest possible degree" (Lucretius, 2007, p. 43). Atoms shift course through a "swerve."

Not only is the swerve or the clinamen relevant to cosmology, it is also relevant to the way plagues begin: by sheer chance. A virus is born—perhaps in one species—and then jumps to another species. Rats, bats and monkeys have been known to carry viruses that have jumped species. There is something about the way in which viruses jump species that results in plagues in human beings. Serres, (2001) in *The Birth of Physics,* goes into much detail about what the clinamen, or the swerve suggests and makes connections to modern-day physics. Lucretius' work has been treated rather dismissively by modern-day scientists—and philosophers—because he is thought to engage in mere "poetry" (Serres, 2001, p. 21). Serres stresses that poetry and philosophy are as important as physics in attempting to understand the world around us. Part of Serres' project, in fact, is to integrate poetry, philosophy, literature and science. And this could be the reason why Serres' work tends to be marginalized among philosophers and scientists—who do not engage in interdisciplinary work. However, there is a richness that philosophers or scientists miss when they dismiss intellectual work that crosses disciplines. Philosophers—like Camus—who do literary fiction as philosophy—tend to be dismissed as well because philosophers generally speaking do not feel that literary fiction is a form of philosophy.

In the previous chapter of this book, it was emphasized that one of Camus' main philosophical concepts is that of the absurd. But for Camus, the absurd was couched in a world of indifference. Serres also discusses the notion of the absurd but here—in the realm of physics—it is used in the context of chance occurrences in cosmology. Serres (2001) comments that the clinamen "is an absurdity" (p. 21) He goes on to say that the clinamen is

> A logical absurdity, since it is introduced without a justification, the cause of Itself before being the cause of all things; [what philosophers would later call the prime mover usually attributed to the concept of God] a geometrical absurdity, in that the definition that Lucretius gives is incomprehensible. (pp. 21-22)

In essence, the clinamen symbolizes chance, or a throw of the dice—if you will. Chance occurrences—like the birth of life-forms—come out of nowhere. Lucretius' text suggests—that the birthing the world is by chance. This remarkable idea—the clinamen, or the swerve—was then later discussed by Epicurus. Althusser (2006) explains:

"Epicurus tells us that, before the formation of the world, an infinity of atoms were falling parallel to each other in the void.... This implies that, before the formation of the world, there was nothing." (p. 169)

Epicurus claims that the atom swerves from a parallel path to "encounter"— as Althusser (2006) suggests—another atom—what Lucretius called a "blow." Althusser suggests that an atom has an "encounter" with another atom—and—" from encounter to encounter, a pile-up of atoms occurs and the birth of the world" (p. 169) unfolds. It is notable that Althusser's book is titled *Philosophy of The Encounter*. Althusser (2006) suggests that these encounters are "aleatory," meaning that that they are "pure" "contingency" (p. 169). Further, Althusser states that behind aleatory encounters of atoms no "[m]eaning" "cause" "end" [r]eason" or "[u]nreason" (pp. 168-169) can be determined.

Leibniz—much later in the history of philosophy— poses the famous question: why is there something rather than nothing? Neither Epicurus or Lucretius will say that a God (or prime mover) created the world. However, Leibniz counters this by declaring that the world is wholly determined by God. Liebniz (2020) in *Discourse on Metaphysics* claims: "God wills everything" (p. 12). "God does nothing out of order" (p. 11). Further Leibniz states that "everything conforms to the universal order. This is so true that, not only does nothing absolutely irregular happen in the world, but one cannot even feign such a thing" (p. 11). Liebniz often compares God to a geometer. When one thinks of geometry, one thinks of grids, symmetry, smooth lines, even spaces. However, there are other kinds of geometries. James Gleick (1987) tells us that for Mandelbrot, geometry looks very different from, say, Liebniz. Gleick (1987) states that for Mandelbrot

"Clouds are not spheres.... Mountains are not cones. Lightning does not travel in a straight line. The new geometry mirrors a universe that is rough, not rounded, scabrous, not smooth. It is a geometry of the pitted, pocked, and broken up, the twisted, tangled and intertwined" (p. 94).

For Mandelbrot, these "irregularities" ironically are, in fact, "regular" (p. 98). Schrodinger, Gleick tells us, thought that "irregularity [was] a building block of life" (p. 300). Thus, for Mandelbrot and Schrodinger, there is a kind of structure in non-structure. Take the case of Lornenz's strange attractors. Gleick (1987) points out that "the deepest problems in nonlinear systems" are what are called strange attractors. What is seemingly chaotic, is in fact "patterned"; "the hidden structures of a system... otherwise [seem] patternless" (p. 153). Thus, according to some modern scientists—like Mandelbrot and Schrodinger and others—Leibniz got it wrong. There are things that occur in the universe that are "irregular" while simultaneously have self-organizing patterns. When one applies this to the occurrence of plagues and pandemics, this makes some sense. Viruses seemingly come out of nowhere, jump species, have irregularities (mutations) but simultaneously have patterns (i.e., the covid virus has a recognizable structure of pattern).

Leibniz felt that God did everything for a reason; that the cause of the universe is deterministic, geometric and orderly. For Liebniz, God "does everything for the best, and that nothing can harm those who love him" (p. 10). Liebniz states "that God permits it, and not that he wills it, although he concurs with it... because he knows to draw from it a greater good" (p. 12). Leibniz' deterministic views are scientifically wrong. Nothing is pre-determined. If God punishes those who do not love him, who needs a God like that? Applied to the covid catastrophe—Leibniz' position falls apart. He encourages a blame the victim mentality—very much like what Camus' Father Paneloux said about those who deserved to get the plague because they engaged in evil. It is astounding—as a chaplain—that the more popular of these viewpoints is that of Father Paneloux and Leibnez. People often ask: what did I do to deserve this illness? I must have done something wrong; I'm being punished by God. Many patients who are dying from covid say things like, "it's God's will, God has a plan—I am too ignorant to understand that plan—and it's all for the best." Or they will say, "There must be a reason that the disease got the better of me; only God knows that reason, it is part of the divine plan." Or, dying patients will say things like "I wouldn't have known happiness had I not suffered, there is a reason for suffering, it balances out the world." These kinds of statements are so entrenched in the popular consciousness that it alarms.

The majority of patients I have cared for have never read or studied Camus, for that matter. The patients whom I care for are mostly under-educated and come from lower socio-economic rural farming communities. Not that farmers do not read—I do not, in any way mean to essentialize—but the patients that I have cared for, counseled and ministered to, have not read Camus or Leibniz. What I think these patients tend to do is repeat what they hear at church; most tend to read the bible literally, not metaphorically. As a chaplain, my job is certainly not to get into theological disputations with patients; my job as a chaplain is certainly not to preach or teach, for that matter. My job is to serve as a holding environment—emotionally—in the Winnicottian (2005) sense. My job is to allow those who are suffering—to suffer—and not interfere with their belief systems. But it is amazing to me, how many patients sound as if they are reciting Leibniz, even though never having read him. Somehow, a deterministic world view—that God's will be done, that God has a plan—is easier to think, than a view that allows for chance occurrences, or to think that there is no God at all. It is more difficult to think in a Lucretian manner, that the clinamen, or the swerve is without cause or reason.

If one takes the Leibnizian view to heart—that this is the best of all possible worlds and God "does everything for the best" (p. 12), I would wonder—again—what kind of God would kill millions of people via covid-19, say? Certainly, this must be a cruel God. A six year old child who dies from covid—or cancer, or any other disease—because God wills it, is not a God that is good. And for those like Bertrand Russell, this is the basis for atheism. What kind of God would allow this cruelty? After witnessing the horrors of world wars, Russell wrote *Why I am Not a Christian*.

> When you come to look into this argument from design[that God has a plan] it is a most astonishing thing that people can believe that this world... should be the best that omnipotence and omniscience have been able to produce in millions of years. I really cannot believe it. Do you think that, if you were granted omnipotence and omniscience and millions of years in which to perfect your world, you could produce nothing better than the Ku Klux Klan or the Fascists? (Russell, 1957, p. 10)

If God really was all good (all knowing and everywhere present) would plagues and pandemics be willed by God? Seemingly chance happenings—say, of plagues and pandemics, some argue—are really pre-determined (but we are ignorant of God's will) for only God knows the grand scheme of things. Poincare (1914), in his *Science and Method,* states "chance is only the measure of our ignorance" (p. 65). Whether things happen because they were already pre-ordained, or pre-determined, whether they seemingly happen by chance—human beings cannot possibly understand God's plan. God's will be done.

Nietzsche (1989)—in his *Beyond Good and Evil*—argued that this kind of moralizing, i.e. Ponciare and Leibniz, is, in actuality, immoral, for words like (good and evil) serve only to justify evil for the sake of some hidden good we are too ignorant to understand. This is why Nietzsche famously calls for the revaluation of values. God is Dead, Nietzsche says, because morality is immoral. It is important to note that Nietzsche's father was a minister for whom he had no great love; or perhaps he both loved and hated him. These, of course are speculative claims. But it is no accident that much of Nietzsche's writings are criticisms of Christianity. Much of Nietzsche's criticisms of religion are perhaps veiled criticisms of his father. Nietzsche's (1896)*Thus Spoke Zarathustra* was intended –perhaps—a corrective to the hypocrisy of Christianity.

Anselms' (1968) proof for the existence of God, a theological geometry, if you will, is another example of determinism. Anselm's (1968) answer to the one who doubts that God created existence remarks that the fool has not understood what he has heard. The fool, is the one who questions God's existence.

The need to have a "reason" a "cause" and "meaning" for everything that happens in the world is rather curious. But Lucretius and Epicurus thought differently. For them there was no reason or cause for anything. All is was sheer chance. As opposed to these aleatory happenings, C.S. Peirce (1955)—suggests that Democritus—an ancient pre-Socratic philosopher—engages in a "strict necessitarianism" (p. 325)—that the world came to be out of necessity— not because of God, but because atoms—or "the impact of matter" (p. 324). Democritus' point of view was at loggerheads with both Lucretius and Epicurus. C.C. W. Taylor (2010) reports that Democritus—among others like Parmenides and Leucippus—all argued in necessitarian fashion. One Stobaeus, states "Parmenides and Democritus say that everything happens by necessity, which is the same as fate, justice, providence, and the creator" (p. 93). This is notable because this is one of the few early fragments that makes direct connections between determinism and fate. If something is fated or driven by "providence" we have another whole host of problems. To say that divine providence was the cost of man-made catastrophes, is a way to exonerate those who are guilty of crimes against humanity, for instance. Countering this position, there is nothing—according to Marx, say, that is pre-ordained, or pre-determined. As Marx (1967) emphasized—people make history; history does not simply sweep people up the torrent of a magical force of Spirit—as Hegel (1977) would have put it. For Hegel (1977) history creates; people are swept into the future because Spirit determines history, not people. The eclipse of human agency has grave consequences especially in light of the Holocaust. And it is this that Hannah Arendt (2006) drove home in her work around the Eichmann trial. Again, I have written extensively about these issues previously so I will not belabor the point here (Morris, 2001).

One of the most important things to learn from Foucault—generally speaking—is that history can happen otherwise. The making of history and even the archiving of history is completely and utterly arbitrary. Spirit, God, the gods, fate, a pre-determined universe, make little sense—according to

Foucault—especially as we begin to understand that even the archiving of these events is done willy-nilly.

In the context of covid-19, there is no reason that this pandemic had to happen. But it did. The shifting and changing of the pandemic, it's intensification and trajectory—has been made worse due to our underestimation of its virility and power. The neglect of the unvaccinated have, indeed, made things worse; more and more variants are to come. If every human being on the globe got vaccinated—which is a statistical improbability—perhaps multiple variants would not have emerged. But there is no way to know this.

Like Michel Serres and Althusser, Alain Badiou (2009) brings the clinamen back into the conversation. Badiou turns the discussion differently. Badiou claims that the point of the clinamen is to disappear. Badiou (2009) states

> The clinamen is outside time, it does not appear in the chain of effects. All effects are subject to law. The clinamen has neither past… nor future (there is no more trace of it) nor present (it has neither a place nor a moment). It takes place only in order to disappear, *it is its very own disappearance* [italics in original]. (p. 62)

This Houdini-like nature of the clinamen—that it "is its very own disappearance" (Badiou, 2009, p. 62) is rather curious. How can something so substantial—and yet so aleatory—just disappear? Into what? Why? Where did it go? Does the clinamen go back into the void with the rest of the atoms? We would hope that if the point of the clinamen is to disappear, so too the virus and its variants will also disappear. However, we see no sign of that at this present historical juncture. But who knows what tomorrow will bring?

Turbulence

Michel Serres (1983), in his book *Hermes: Literature, Science, Philosophy,* writes about the clinamen and connects it to the concept of turbulence. This notion became the basis for what today is called "strange attractors" in contemporary science (Gleick, 1987, p. 4). Serres argues that the clinamen is another name for the beginning(s) of turbulence. Serres (1983) explains:

> In nature, living beings are born from flows. And these flows are laminar, their laminae parallel to one another; the declination is the tiniest angle necessary and sufficient to produce turbulence. (pp. 101-102)

It was Epicurus—Serres points out—who used the phrase "[o]f the angle in the atom" (p. 102). It is this angle, this deviation from the parallel laminae that set off the "blow" of atoms crashing against atoms, creating existence.

Turbulence, a word often associated with chaos and complexity theory, describes the universe not as a geometrical grid, but signifies strange patterns especially in weather. Weather patterns—are becoming more and more extreme due to global warming. In fact, weather patterns are creating their own weather systems, scientist tell us. Lightning and tornadoes, heat rising in Oregon, floods devastating China, snow in Atlanta Georgia, Siberia self-generating fires, buildings collapsing in South Florida are due to rising sea levels are inter-related patterns of turbulence.

Serres (1983) points out that as early as Cicero, the notion of turbulence had been discussed. Serres (1983) states that "In the *De Finibus,* Cicero wrote that *atomorum turbulenta concursio,* that is, atoms meet in and by turbulence" (p. 24). It is important to point out—as David Webb and William Ross (2001) tell us, that "The French term *tourbillon* that Serres adopts to denote... turbulent yet stable structure that forms in fluid flow [also] translated... as 'vortex'" (p. 26).

Likewise, chaos theorists and those who have done work on fractals have pointed out, too, that there is also order in the universe; that fractals have patterns. But on a phenomenological and more philosophical level, it feels as if—right now at this juncture in history—we are living through utter and complete turbulence; we are living in complete chaos as global warming—in the intersection of the pandemic—rage. Some suggest that the pandemic is part and parcel of global warming, that it, in other words, might be an effect of global warming.

It is interesting that in Serres' work he often makes references to plagues and pandemics. Recall, Richard Jenkyns (2001) mentions—when introducing Serres' work on *The Birth of Physics*—that around 430 BCE Lucretius' book ended as a plague ravaged Athens. Serres (2001) states "[v]iolence is still, always, within physics. The germ atoms wreak havoc on Athens, the last survivors killing each other" (p. 159). Serres (2001) states "the plague returns" (p. 158). In *Hermes* Serres (1983) states "[a]nd here again is the plague. It is always the same sequence of events: an epidemic becomes pandemic in proportions, if not to say a pandemonium" (p. 100). Later Serres states "[t]he law is the plague.... Everything falls to zero, a complete lack of information, the nothingness of knowledge, non-existence" (p. 100).

Serres (2001) compares a plague of atoms to Hiroshima for two reasons, I believe. One is that atom bombs are akin to plagues because like plagues, atom bombs cause death and utter decimation. Serres also points out that the plague that ravaged Athens in 430 ended up in "the last survivors killing each other" (p. 159). Like atom bombs, plagues turn people against one another in a Hobbesian war of all-against-all. During covid-19, there has been an uptick in gun violence, domestic violence—a kind of Hobbesian all-against-all. Parents kill their children; children kill the parents; citizens overthrow their own governments—or attempt to, in the case of the January 6th insurrection that occurred at the United States Capitol. The schools are in complete and utter chaos during this third year of the pandemic; high school students in New York City, in Chicago and in some places in California are staging walk-outs because of unsafe conditions in schools due to the virus. Parents and teachers are at odds whether to continue remote learning or go back into the classroom; omicron, the latest variant, has come on seemingly out of nowhere and now is creating complete turmoil in hospitals, businesses, colleges and universities, meat packing factories and so forth. Vaccines do not seem to be as efficacious as scientists had predicted; many are still dying from the virus, some have even been vaccinated. In Europe, a more virulent strain of omicron has been detected in some 50 people and is expected to be yet the next wave of the pandemic that might evade vaccine protection altogether. We are living in an age of turbulence, unlike anything we have seen in one-hundred years. This is a curriculum of turbulence on a grand scale. There is nothing in our education(s) that have prepared us for what we are experiencing because of covid.

Noise

In Serres' (1995) *Genesis* he bases his ideas on what is called information theory and cybernetics. Genevieve James and James Nielson—the translators of Serres' (1995) *Genesis* point out—the word noise—as Serres' uses it in the book—does not have the same meaning as it used by information theorists. James and Nielson translate the concept noise to mean "strife, contention" (p. 141). This clarification is important. Serres (1995) makes connections between noise—as a metaphor for strife and turbulence. For example, Serres (1995) states: "The *noise* intermittence and turbulence—quarrel and racket—this sea *noise* is the originating rumor and murmuring, the original hate. We hear it on the high seas" (p. 14). Two things of note here. Pre-Socratic philosopher Empedocles described the world a kind of turmoil between love and hate. The myth of Empedocles is that he tossed himself into a volcano, perhaps in an attempt to quell hate or to experience hate. There is no telling what the myth of Empedocles means, however. The point here being that perhaps Serres had Empedocles in mind when he uses the word "hate" in the context of noise and turbulence.

Secondly, Serres served in the navy during World War II. He uses sea metaphors—perhaps—because of his service in the navy. The sea can become quite turbulent. When one is sailing in the middle of the sea during a storm—a good metaphor for that experience is that the sea is full of hate. Hate is a kind of turbulence and unease that makes one queasy.

Serres (1995) states that "the cosmos appears turbulent to us... that it is fractal, intermittent" (p. 109). Fractals, recall, exhibit patterns. The cosmos—for Serres—exhibits both chaos and order. And this, too, is what the pre-Socratic philosopher Empedocles was suggesting—that the world is both orderly (love) and chaotic (hate). However, Serres (1995) is in no way cutting the cosmos into two: love and hate, or order and chaos. In fact, things are much more complex than that. Throughout Serres' work, and in *Genesis*—especially—he states "I am attempting to extricate myself from the hell of dualism. Utterly pure rationality is a myth" (p. 131). Rationality in philosophy—since at least Plato—has taken nuance out of philosophy. Donna Haraway (1997), like Serres, calls for the "implosion" (p. 12) of dualisms as everything is interconnected to everything in complex webs. The postmodern project writ- large is, indeed, a battle against dualisms, bifurcations, simplifications and so forth. A curriculum of "implosion" is one where everything caves in on itself, things are interwoven and webbed in detailed and complex interconnections. This is why, when the disciplines split apart during the late 19th century, problems in academe got only worse. The separation of disciplines was the beginning of turf warfare in academe—something about which Serres' rails against. Serres has suggested that the university is a battlefield; university politics are, indeed, war-games where nobody wins. Serres' is a Renaissance philosopher—whereby all disciplines should be inter-connected, "imploded"—to use Haraway's term. But cross-disciplinary studies is considered suspect—still—for more conservative academicians. Groundbreaking and paradigm shifting work is currently being done in the humanities—both in comparative literature and in curriculum studies. Philosophers like Serres, Derrida, Avital Ronell and Judith Butler, have found their homes not in philosophy departments, but in departments of comparative literature and curriculum studies. The covid-19 catastrophe demands the integration of academic disciplines to attempt to cope with all of the social and scientific problems that we are facing. Life and death issues need to be studied by an entire array of scholars and clinicians: the health-humanities, hospital chaplaincy, public health, social work, bioethics, political scientists, philosophers, psychoanalysts, psychologists, psychiatrists, counselors—as well as experts in the medical profession—and educationists, generally speaking—if we are to ever get a handle on this virus. If anything, today—more than ever—we need to work together in cross-disciplinary fashion—in what Haraway (1997) calls an "implosion" (p. 12) of disciplines if we are to become better equipped—educationally—to cope with what is happening to us. If anything, we need to begin to think about *interfering*—as Serres might contend- with and creating turbulence in the very educational systems we have inherited—in order to overturn stale paradigms that are keeping us from understanding the present moment, the past and the future, if we have a future at all.

Interference—a metaphor drawn from information theory—is another way Serres (1995) writes about noise. Noise is, in fact, interference. Serres (1995) states:

> Noise is parasitical, like interference, it follows the logic of the parasite, a very tiny thing, an insufficient reason, a cause without consequences at times, which may vanish to the left of the dovetail. (p. 57)

Here, Serres' concept of noise resonates with Badiou's (2009) take on the clinamen. Recall, Badiou says that the strange thing about the clinamen is "the vanishing term" (p. 62) "*it is its own disappearance*" (p. 62). Likewise, Serres suggests that noise (like the clinamen) is a "very tiny thing" that "may vanish" (p. 57). Let us hope that covid-19 "vanishe[s] to the left of the dovetail" (Serres, 1995, p. 57). Who knows what our future holds? Either we will vanish, or the pandemic will. Or, we will not vanish nor will the pandemic. What part does chance play in the disappearance of anything?

The Vanishing of Concepts

Deleuze and Guattari (1994) suggest that philosophy concerns the creation of concepts. Not only that, philosophy is also about the disappearance of concepts over time. They discuss the importance of the way in which—what they call "the plane of immanence" (p. 41)—or "the ground of philosophy" (p. 41) "the foundation on which it creates it concepts" (p. 41)—"vanish[es]" (p. 42). Just as the clinamen vanishes, so, too, do philosophical concepts. Deleuze and Guattari (1994) state

> The plane of immanence is like a section of chaos and acts like a sieve. In fact, chaos is characterized less by the absence of determinations than by the infinite speed with which they [the creation of concepts] take place and vanish. (p. 42)

Similarly, Serres (1995) similarly suggests that—in the context of the creation of concepts and their disappearance—meaning "vanishes" too. He states "meaning vanishes from the place that I call forth. It is an entirely blank place" (p. 43). That "blank place" is not dissimilar to the void—a concept about which Lucretius writes. The void is also—for Serres—akin to death. Serres (1995) states "Hopelessly, I am attempting to open up Pandora's little casket" (p. 4). Death is the void; it is the vanishing point. The attempt to define death or the void—that "blank place" is no easy task. In fact, Serres (1995) warns: "The bottom always falls out of the quest for the elementary" (p. 3). Any "elementary" explanation of death—i.e. that the heart stops beating, for example—comes up short against the complexities of what death actually is—which is beyond our understanding and beyond representation and signification.

The Pandemic

Philosophical concepts are useful in making connections through metaphor, opening portals of meaning, or the lack thereof. However, the discourse of disjointed metaphors (clinamen, turbulence, noise) do not make for a philosophical *system*. Philosophical systems—in the Enlightenment traditions of, say, Kant and Hegel—are counter to what it is that Serres' is doing in his work on philosophy. Serres' philosophical oeuvre is in no way systematic. In fact, he swerved—to use Lucretius' concept—out of classical philosophy. Serres' is more interested in fragmented ideas, disjointed concepts. It is difficult to piece together—in a smooth whole—Serres' disjunctions and discontinuities because they do not fit into any recognizable schema. Serres' work mirrors the way in which experience unfolds: in a disjointed, confusing, disorganized fashion. Is this not the way most experience the way in which this current pandemic is unfolding? All seems chaotic, ever-changing. Deleuze and Guattari (1994) comment on the fragmentary nature of doing philosophy:

> Philosophical concepts are fragmentary wholes that are not aligned with one another so that they fit together, because their edges do not match up. They are not pieces of a jigsaw puzzle but rather the outcomes of throws of the dice. (p. 35)

Stephane Mallarme (cited in, Marty 2018, np) famously declared: *"A Throw of the Dice Will Never Abolish Chance.* James Gleick (1987) says of cosmology that" [i]n the presence of nonlinearity, a perturbation [what Serres would call turbulence] can feed on itself until it dies away" (pp. 193-194). A "perturbation" is akin to turbulence, say, when flying. One can feel turbulence in an airplane and one can also feel when it "dies away."

The way one experiences the present is hard to say because of the fluidity of time. The way one experiences living through a pandemic is akin to an upheaval in the flow of things. The way that the pandemic gets represented in words and concepts change—as the pandemic changes. Moreover, the way in which historians will recall these events will also change over time. Historians will re-present the past through the lens of their present. The way in which this event gets archived—now—will effect the way in which historians re-present the past. Karl Popper (1990) puts it this way:

> Our very understanding of the world changes the condition of the changing world; and so do our wishes, our preferences, our hypothesis, our theories. Even our erroneous theories change the world. (p. 17)

In other words, the way we think about the nature of change in the world, changes the world about which we think. The way we write about and represent the changing world, changes the very world about which we write.

Against this ever-changing and fluid relationship between the one who archives and the way in which the very archivization changes the way we think about what gets represented, in the context of the current pandemic, any effort to document these ever-changing interrelationships between the writer and what gets written is always already beyond our understanding.

In other words, covid-19 cannot be reduced to simple terms. Serres—in connection with Lucretius —connects concepts like the clinamen, turbulence and noise with "pandemonium" (1995, p. 4) and with plagues. Indeed, what we are currently living through seems like "pandemonium." It is important to note that Serres died before the advent of covid-19 but he had studied plagues historically and understood them in historical terms. In a book titled *Rome: The Book of Foundations,* Serres (1991) writes extensively on plagues. Serres (1991) says:

> In the state of the plague nobody knows who has the plague, and nobody knows how to decide who has it and who doesn't, who carries and spreads it. In the state of war we are all Horatius or Fabius, plebeian or Veian, all in uniform; but in the state of plague we can no longer distinguish those who are for or against, near or far, known or unknown. (p. 199)

As we enter the third year of Covid-19—this current and horrific pandemic— it seems that things are getting worse. The way in which we experience this pandemic is not unlike what Serres describes above. "Nobody knows who has the plague, and nobody knows how to decide who has it and who doesn't" (p. 199). Who is friend and who is foe? Who has covid, who does not? How does one maneuver this terrain without becoming paranoid.

Tests for Covid-19 are far from accurate, positives results could be false negatives; negative results could be wrong. The efficacy of the vaccines are not what the scientists thought; however, for many being vaccinated means avoiding being hospitalized. Healthy people have gotten fully vaccinated but can still fall ill with Covid. ICUs are at capacity in many parts of the country, in many countries around the globe. Everyone is at risk; but it seems that too many are complacent. Every time we think that we have turned a corner on the pandemic it seems to come back even worse.

During the 1918 flu pandemic just when people thought the pandemic was over, they flooded the streets thinking that they were free from turmoil and death. It was at that point that people began vanishing in droves. The difference during the 1918 flu pandemic was that someone could get sick in the morning and be dead by nightfall. Soldiers carried the flu with them to war—without knowing it—and spread the flu across Europe. But even though today we have lockdowns in many countries and strict rules of entering countries, it has not stopped the pandemic from killing scores of people. Who knows how long covid will be here; some scientists think it is here to stay. That is a sobering thought.

The clinamen, that tiny swerve, that atom, that germ, that blow—as Lucretius called it—created life-forms, so Lucretius thought. Life-forms were created by sheer chance, in momentary collisions of atoms. Similarly, it only takes one "germ atom," as Serres put it, to end life. One "germ atom" and five minutes with someone who has covid is enough to make an entire room full of people sick. We have to fear everyone; and perhaps it is this fear and resultant paranoia that is driving so much violence—especially in the United States where guns are readily available.

In the context of ancient Rome—during the plague—Serres (1991) states: "I meet the enemy; if he doesn't bring me the plague, he could become my brother, whereas if my neighbor is an active carrier of the epidemic I stop being his friend. The adversary could be benign: I no longer know who my neighbor is." (p. 199-200). Do we not feel similarly today? Who is friend? Who is foe? Who is neighbor? Who is enemy? Which students in the classroom are unvaccinated and covid positive? How many students have covid? There is little contact tracing or transparency in classrooms. Sometimes entire schools are shutting down; while some colleges and universities are pretending that all is well with the world. Nobody is told who has covid; the teaching continues in contaminated classroom; unventilated and contaminated air-flows are killing teachers and those who are vulnerable. And yet we carry on as if nothing is happening. And yet, everybody knows that something is afoot—something so unbelievable and frightening that we cannot get hold of what is happening.

Epidemiologists, infectious disease specialists and public health experts have been warning—for a long time—that an airborne virus would come to our shores. No one listened. The clinamen, turbulence and noise—three concepts Serres focuses much of his work on—are metaphors for the way in which many of us are experiencing living through covid. All it takes is contact with one infected person in the grocery store, on a college committee, at the gas station to become infected. It is a game of chance, a throw of the dice. It is madness.

A throw of the dice. A game of chance. Covid, however, is no game. For some, it is life or death. All of our schooling, all of our training, all of our disciplines come up short against something as terrifying and grave as this pandemic. Although we know from history that there have been many pandemics before us—as Serres knew well—it seems that we are always-already in denial: Plagues are a thing of the past. It won't happen here. *But it is happening here; it is happening now.* Nietzsche (1974) famously asked: "What did I really experience? What happened in me and around me at the time" (p. 253)? What did I really experience as I witnessed—first-hand—the dying, the dead, the body-bags. What did I really experience when I got sick from covid the first time, the second time, and perhaps maybe once again? I am still too close to the situation at hand—as we all are—to answer Nietzsche's question. I I have seen things I wish that I had never seen. I experienced the unthinkable, the non-conceptual. Maurice Blanchot (1995) writes: "We are on the edge of disaster without being able to situate it in the future: it is rather always already past, and yet we are on the edge or under the threat" (p. 1). This pandemic, has indeed, put us "on the edge of disaster"; Perhaps it will take decades, a lifetime, perhaps I will never understand what I have witnessed or what I have experienced during these years of the pandemic.

There is no way to contain the grief of those who lost loved ones to this pandemic. The day I witnessed a nurse crying in the hallway of the ICU; I was overcome with an utter hopelessness and speechlessness. The chaplain is supposed to be there for hospital staff. I did not know how to be there anymore. Respiratory therapists—in hopeless resignation—went about their jobs as if in a factory, one intubation followed by an extubation; another intubation followed by an extubation, over and over again. Many of those put on ventilators never recovered; the ventilator in the first year of the pandemic was a symbol of death.

Nietzsche (2009) states: "To have something *behind* [italics in the original] you that you should never have wanted, something that constitutes a nodal point in the destiny of humanity—and from then on to have it *on top of you*! [italics in the original]... It almost crushes you" (p. 70). The pandemic, however, is not yet "behind" us; it continues creating a crushing weight of memories. Gloves, debris, the leftovers of a medical disaster all over the floor; leaving the corpse to the custodians of the dead. The undertakers. The morgue. The phone call. The screams. What are worse are the silences, when the telephone line goes dead. Am I the angel of death? The chaplain has always been figured as the angel of death historically. But what does that mean? Michel Serres (1993) in his book titled *Angels: A Modern Myth* points out that the angel of death is an archetypal image that spans ancient Greek culture through the birth of Islam and beyond. Serres (1993) tells us that the angel of death or,

> The psychopomp angel, the angel that accompanies the souls of the dead and after death, appears in the polytheist traditions of Greece (where the role is played by Hermes), Egypt and Rome and in the Monotheist religions of Judaism, Christianity and Islam. (p. 124)

Chaplains are messengers of death. This is a heavy burden. But where is God in all of this? Still, the ones who are left behind believe that God has a plan, that the death of their loved one was part of their destiny. Nietzsche (2008) in *The Twilight of Idols* exclaims: "Hence their astounding notion of 'God'... The last, thinnest, emptiest [concept] is put, as cause in itself" (p. 18). And again, I ask, what kind of God would allow for so many deaths? As Nietzsche points out God is but a concept; the concept God is not a reality. But religious people believe that God is reality, not a concept. In *Ecce Homo*, Nietzsche (2009) exclaimed: "What is the point of those mendacious, morality's *ancillary* [italics in original] concepts 'soul', 'spirit' 'free will' 'God', if not to bring about humanity's physiological ruin?" (p. 63). Nietzsche argued that these concepts serve to pacify. Nietzsche claimed that concepts like God and prayer, make people stop thinking altogether. Prayer, for Nietzsche, was a way to avoid thinking the *unthinkable*.

Television—as we know it in the United States—and especially the news is highly controlled and contained. Judith Butler (2020) remarks that "[t]he public sphere is constituted in part by what cannot be said and what cannot be shown" (p. xvii). TV—and those who have the power to control the images that stream into our living rooms—sanitize and contain the "unsayable" and "what cannot be shown" because what cannot be shown—or spoken about—cannot be contained.

Jean-Luc Nancy (1997) says "In other words, there is no longer any sense of the world" (p. 4). Or, he puts it this way: "this *end of the sense of the world* [italics in the original]... is the *end of the world of sense*" [italics in the original] (p. 5). That we cannot make sense of the world of or make sense of sense is what it feels like to live through a pandemic. Without a visceral engagement with the real, the public lacks a sense of what is happening in the world; the general public lacks a visceral sense of the pandemic as it is seen from the ICU. Ongoing denial and disengagement from the real is partly what is killing people. The unvaccinated—still—three years into covid—do not believe that this pandemic is real. The Stoic philosopher Seneca (2018) cites Epicurus who stated "Rehearse for death," "it's a great thing to learn how to die." (p. 2). But there is no way to "rehearse for death" and no one can actually "learn how to die." Especially today. Death is everywhere present; but it is seemingly absent from public awareness. It seems that far too many are complacent or just do not think the pandemic is real.

Perhaps if the public actually saw, sensed, and experienced what hospital workers have lived through, what families have gone through losing loved ones to covid, things might be different. But remarkably—even when families do see what is happening to their loved ones as they are dying, hooked up to machines behind glass-enclosed walls—they do not believe that covid is real. To see something is not necessarily to believe it. Derrida (2007), remarked before he died, that he did not learn how to die; nor did he learn how to live. His words counter those of the stoic Seneca.

The Unbearable Story of Covid

Covid is a story that is unbearable. Metaphors and philosophical concepts, the words of the poets—somehow open portals otherwise not available over against the literalness of blood, dirty rags, corpses and code blues. Making connections between the metaphors such as the clinamen, turbulence and noise are not easy. Why don't you just tell me your story? Critics might say. Why use all these difficult metaphors? Why draw on obscure philosophies? I answer: literal descriptions of death, of code blues, of ventilators, of feet turning blue, of screaming mothers who have lost a loved one—are not enough. The literal leaves me cold. The literal leaves us without a way to think through—in more philosophical, conceptual, educational terms—what we are living through. In a way, we need a different language to talk about what is literally happening to us. Otherwise, we are stuck in the literal, the everyday and learn little from that. Ordinary language keeps us turning in circles, gets us stuck in the status quo of language and lacks deeper understanding, or even the understanding that we lack the understanding to comprehend what is happening.

There are no precedents for these kinds of stories, the stories of covid. Even if I wrote a book of verbatim stories from hospital beds, that would not allow portals to open so that we might think otherwise. Thinking otherwise means thinking through other ways of being. We do not have a narrative for covid; for covid doesn't happen in narrative form in the first place. Covid is a pandemic without a narrative. One might argue that stories are narratives. In some ways, yes they are. But in more profound ways stories of covid are not narratives but disjointed, turbulent silences that are beyond signification.

Things are indeed turbulent; we are falling into an unending void. And it takes one small mistake, one step the wrong way to get infected, sick and possibly die. The clinamen is at hand; it is that swerve, that tiny swerve the wrong way, crashing into a deadly virus, unknown to us because it is invisible. We are living in an invisible world of enemies. It is nearly impossible to articulate at a phenomenological level what it feels like to live through a pandemic such as this. And yet that is what this book attempts to do: to dig into that impossible phenomenological task at hand. Still, the task remains impossible. I recall as an undergraduate student reading a paper by Thomas Nagel called "What is it like to be a bat?" At the time, I thought it was a rather humorous critique of the impossibilities of empathy. Nagel's answer to his seemingly ridiculous question is: how should I know? I am not a bat. But Nagel's question is not humorous now, in the context of the covid pandemic. What it is like to die from covid? What is it like to witness someone dying from covid? What is it like to talk to a mother screaming on the phone when told of the bad news that her son just died from covid? Even as a chaplain—I must say—I do not know what it is like to be on the other end of that telephone. I do not know what it is like to be that mother who hears the terrible news. Still, a limited form of empathy is necessary in order that we do not become cold and callous. Those who become totally numb to the work of chaplaincy should quit. When feelings leave you, you can no longer have even a limited sense of empathy for the Other.

This covid pandemic is a deep psychic wound. Serres (2012) explains that

> One of the epidemics whose ravages, for centuries, decimated our ancestors so often, the plague... then broke out in Selinunte. The people of that city, neighboring Agrigentum, called for help from he whose theory and practices controlled, they believed, the elements. Empedocles observed then that the plague was spreading from the surrounding springs and backwaters. (p. 72)

The legend of Empedocles is that he stopped the spread of plague by "draining the swamps" (p. 72), preventing the waters from killing people. Serres cites Empedocles who declares: "To cure men and women of the plague I vanquished, through love, the hate of the foul waters" (cited in Serres, 2012, pp. 72-73). The legend of Empedocles serves as a psychological balm. But the Balm of Gilead—in any form—only serves to gloss over the horrors at hand.

Derrida (2001) writes about the loss of Louis Marin, a well-known figure in French intellectual circles who died in 1993. A few years later, Derrida would begin suffering from pancreatic cancer; Derrida succumbed to that cancer and died in 2004. Perhaps Derrida intuited his own death to come as his words in the eulogy to Marin sound eerily autobiographical. Derrida (2001) remarks:

> One cannot hold a discourse on the "work of mourning" without taking part in it, without announcing or partaking in... death, and first of all in one's own death. In the announcement of one's own death, which says, in short, "I am dead," "I died"—such as this book lets it be heard —one should be able to say, and I have said this in the past that all work is also the work of mourning. (p. 143)

Even though Derrida died before the outbreak of covid-19, he speaks to today's issues, just as to his own. The death of so many of Derrida's friends—as documented in his book on mourning—is a testimony to those whom Derrida wished to honor. Let my book also be a testament, a testimonial to the dead. Unless we archive the dead, they will disappear from history forever. We must never let our memories disappear; it is through archivization that memory work—in the Freudian sense—becomes historical. Without memory and history, we have no past and no future, for the future is built on the past.

Derrida (1997), writes in *Adieu: To Emmanuel Levinas*:

> For a long time, for a very long time, I've feared having to say *Adieu* to Emmanuel Levinas.... Whom is one addressing at such a moment? And in whose name would one allow oneself to do so? Often those who come forward to speak, to speak publicly thereby interrupting the animated whispering, the secret or intimate exchange that always links one, deep inside, to a friend or master, those who make themselves heard in a cemetery, end up addressing *directly, straight on,* the one who, as we say, is no longer, is no longer living. (p. 1)

The "one who is no longer living," Derrida remarks, is the one who can "no longer respond" (p. 2). This is an important point—especially for Levinas. Response and responsibility—to respond to the Other without any expectation in return—was

Levinas' mantra. To respond to the one who is no longer able to live is the task at hand, here, too.

Serres, Derrida and Levinas are all gone now; they have all died. This book is, in part, a testimony to the works of those upon whom I draw, especially those who have vanished. Thomas Merton is gone; Joan Didion recently died; Louise DeSalvo died, John Gunther is gone, Albert Camus is dead, Anton Boisen is dead. This book is my *Adieu* to all of those who came before me, those who have made my thought possible during these terrible years of covid. Judith Butler (2020) stresses that life is precarious. How to live in a time of precariousness, Butler (2020) asks? I have witnessed more death and dying than anyone should. But this story of covid is not about me: it is, rather, a testimony to the dead.

References

Abraham, N., Torok, M. (1978). *The shell and the kernel.* Chicago, IL: University of Chicago Press.
Abram, D. (1996). *Spell of the sensuous.* New York: Vintage.
Adorno, T. W. (1966/2007). *Negative dialectics.* New York: Continuum.
Adorno, T. W. (2005). *Minima moralia: Reflections on a damaged life.* New York: Verso.
Adorno, T. W. (2008). *Lectures on negative dialectics.* Malden, MA: Polity.
Althusser, L. (2006). *Philosophy of the encounter: Later writings, 1978-1987.* New York: Verso.
Anselm. (1968). *Proslogium.* In Walter Kaufman (Ed.), *Philosophic classics: From Thales to Ockham* (pp. 522–523). Englewood Cliffs, NJ: Prentice Hall.
Arendt, H. (1951). *The origins of totalitarianism.* New York: Schocken.
Arendt, H. (1978). *The life of the mind.* New York: Harcourt Brace & Company.
Arendt, H. (1994). *Essays in understanding 1930-1954: Formation, exile, and totalitarianism.* New York: Schocken Books.
Arendt, H. (2003). *Responsibility and judgment.* New York: Schocken Books.
Arendt, H. (2005). *The promise of politics.* New York: Schocken Books.
Arendt, H. (2006). *Eichmann in Jerusalem: A report on the banality of evil.* New York: Penguin.
Aristotle. (1987). *The Nichomachean ethics* (Transl., J. E. C. Welldon). Buffalo, NY: Prometheus Books.
Aristotle. (1996). *Poetics.* New York: Penguin Classic.
Athanasisus. (335CE/1980). *The life of Antony and the letter to Marcellinus.* Mahwah, NJ: Paulist Press.
Augustine. (1961). *Confessions.* New York: Penguin.

References

Bachelard, G. (2002). *Earth and reveries of will: An essay on the imagination of matter*. Dallas, TX: The Dallas Institute.

Badiou, A. (2009). *Theory of the subject* (Transl., Bruno Bosteels). New York: Continuum.

Balibar, E. (2020). *On universals: Constructing and deconstructing community*. New York: Fordham University Press.

Bateson, G. (2000). *Steps to an ecology of mind*. Chicago: University of Chicago Press.

Behar, R. (1997). *The vulnerable observer: Anthropology that breaks your heart*. Boston, MA: Beacon Press.

Benjamin, W. (1978). A Berlin chronicle. In Peter Demetz (Ed.), *Walter Benjamin: Essays, aphorisms, autobiographical writings* (pp. 3-60). New York: Schocken Books.

Benjamin, W. (1996a). *Selected writings: Volume 4, 1938-1940* (Transl., Edmund Jephcott and others). Cambridge, MA: The Belknap Press of Harvard University Press.

Benjamin, W. (1996b). *The writer of modern life: Essays on Charles Baudelaire*. Cambridge, MA: The Belknap Press of Harvard University Press.

Benjamin, W. (1999). *The arcades project*. Cambridge, MA: Harvard University Press.

Benjamin, W. (2016). *The storyteller: Tales out of loneliness* (Transl., Sam Dolbear, Esther Leslie & Sebastian Truskolaksi). New York: Verso.

Bergson, H. (2015). *Time and free will: An essay on the immediate data of consciousness* (Transl., F. L. Pogson). Mansfield, CT: Martino Publishing.

Bergman, I. (1963). *Winter light*. Director Ingmar Berman. Janus Films.

Bergman, I. (1982). *Fanny and Alexander*. Director Ingmar Bergman. Sandrew Film & Teater.

Blanchot, M. (1995). *The writing of disaster* (Transl., Ann Smock). Lincoln, NE: University of Nebraska Press.

Bloom, A. (2012). *The closing of the American mind*. New York: Simon & Schuster.

Boisen, A. (1952). *The exploration of the inner world: A Study of mental disorder and religious experience*. New York: Harper & Brothers.

Bollas, C. (1986). *The shadow of the object: Psychoanalysis of unthought known*. New York: Columbia University Press.

Bonhoeffer, D. (1937/1995). *The cost of discipleship*. New York: Touchstone.

Bowles, P. (1949/1977). *The sheltering sky*. New York: The Ecco Press/Harper Collins.

Bree, G. (1974). *Camus and Sarte: Crisis and commitment*. London: Caldar & Boyars.

Brentano, F. (1874/1995). *Psychology from an empirical standpoint*. New York: Routledge.

Brodersen, M. (1997). *Walter Benjamin: A biography* (Transl., Malcolm R. Green & Ingrida Ligers). New York: Verso.

Bruner, J. S. (1987). Foreword to the 1987 Edition. In A. R. Luria, *The mind of a mnemonist: A little book about a vast memory* (pp. ix–xix). Cambridge, MA: Harvard University Press.

Burns, K. (2018). How Thomas Merton and Keith Jarrett changed my life. In Jon Sweeney (Ed.), *What am I living for: Lessons from the life and writings of Thomas Merton* (pp. 105-109). Notre Dame, IN: Ave Maria Press.

Butler, J. (1997). *Excitable speech: A politics of the performative*. New York: Routledge.

Butler, J. (2016). *Frames of war: When is life grievable?* New York: Verso.

Butler, J. (2019). *Giving an account of oneself*. New Delhi, India: Dev Publishers & Distributors.

Butler, J. (2020). *Precarious life: The powers of mourning and justice*. New York: Verso.

Camus, A. (1946/1989). *The stranger.* New York: Vintage.
Camus, A. (1948). *The plague* (Transl., Stuart Gilbert). New York: The Modern Library.
Camus, A. (1955/1983). *The myth of Sisyphus* (Transl., Justin O'Brien). New York: Vintage.
Camus, A. (1956/1991). *The rebel: An essay on man in revolt.* New York: Vintage.
Camus, A. (1970). *Albert Camus: Lyrical and critical essays.* New York: Vintage.
Camus, A. (1977). *Youthful writings: Albert Camus.* New York: Vintage.
Camus, A. (1991). *The rebel: An essay on man in revolt.* New York: Vintage.
Camus, A. (1995). *The first man* (Transl., David Hapgood). New York: Alfred A. Knopf.
Camus, A. (2007). *Exile and the kingdom.* New York: Vintage.
Camus, C. (1995). Editor's note. In Albert Camus' *The First Man* (pp. v–viii). New York: Alfred A. Knopf.
Carretto, C. (1964/2002). *Letters from the desert.* New York: Orbis Books.
Carson, R. (1962). *Silent spring.* New York: Houghton Mifflin.
Casey, E. (1998). *The fate of place: A philosophical history.* Berkeley, CA: University of California Press.
Chryssavgis, J. (2008). *In the heart of the desert: The spirituality of the desert fathers and mothers.* Bloomington, IN: World Wisdom.
Deignan, K. (2007). Introduction. In *Thomas Merton, A book of hours* (pp. 15-42). Notre Dame, IN: Sorin Books.
Delancey, C. (2019). Albert Camus: Unfashionable anti-totalitarian. In *Quillett (np). Quillete. com.*
Deleuze, G. (1989). *Cinema 2: The time-image* (Transl., Hugh Tomlinson & Robert Galeta). Minneapolis, MN: University of Minnesota Press.
Deleuze, G., Guattari, F. (1994). *What is philosophy?* (Transl., Hugh Tomlinson & Graham Burchell). New York: Columbia University Press.
Deleuze, G., Guattatri, F. (2000). *Anti-Oedipus: Capitalism and schizophrenia* (Tranls., Robert Hurley, Mark Seem & Helen R. Lane). Minneapolis, MN: The University of Minnesota Press.
Deleuze, G., Guattari. F. (2002). *A thousand plateaus: Capitalism and schizophrenia* (Transl., Brian Massumi). Minneapolis, MN: University of Minnesota Press.
Democritus. (2010). *The Atomists: Leucippus and Democritus. Fragments* (Transl., C.C. W. Taylor). Toronto: University of Toronto Press.
Derrida, J. (1976). *Of grammatology* (Transl., Gayatri Chakravorty Spivak). Baltimore: The Johns Hopkins University Press.
Derrida, J. (1987). *The postcard: From Socrates to Freud and beyond* (Transl., Alan Bass). Chicago, IL: University of Chicago Press.
Derrida, J. (1991). Living on: Border lines. In Peggy Kamuf (Ed.), *A Derrida Reader: Between the blinds* (pp. 257-268). New York: Columbia University Press.
Derrida, J. (1992). *Logomachia: The conflict of the faculties.* Lincoln, NE: University of Nebraska Press.
Derrida, J. (1994). *Specters of Marx: The state of debt, the work of mourning, & the new international.* New York: Routledge.
Derrida, J. (1996). *Archive fever: A Freudian impression* (Transl., Eric Prenowitz). Chicago: University of Chicago Press.

Derrida, J. (1997). *Adieu to Emmanuel Levinas*. Stanford, CA: Stanford University Press.
Derrida, J. (2000). *Of hospitality* (Transl., Rachel Bowlby). Stanford, CA: Stanford University Press.
Derrida, J. (2001). *The work of mourning*. Chicago: University of Chicago Press.
Derrida, J. (2003). Derrida. *The Film*. Directed by Kirby Dick & Amy Ziering Kofman. Zeitgeist Films Ltd.
Derrida, J. (2005). *On touching—Jean-Luc Nancy* (Transl., Christine Irizarry). Stanford, CA: Stanford University Press.
Derrida, J. (2007). *Learning to live finally: An interview with Jean Birnaum* (Transl., Pascale-Anne Brault & Michael Ness). Hoboken, NJ: Melville House Publishing.
DeSalvo, L. (2018). *The house of early sorrows: A memoir in essays*. New York: Fordham University Press.
Descartes, R. (1996). *Discourse on method and meditations on first philosophy*. New Haven, CT: Yale University Press.
Diat, N. (2019). *A time to die: Monks on the threshold of eternal life*. San Francisco, CA: Ignatius Press.
Didion, J. (2005). *The year of magical thinking*. New York: Vintage.
Duigan, J. (1989). *Romero*. Director, John Duigan. Paulist Pictures. Warner Brothers.
Eckhart, M. (1941). *Meister Eckhart*. New York: Harper Perennial.
Ellsberg, R. (2018). On spiritual exploration. In, Jon Sweeney (Ed.), *What am I living for: The life and writings of Thomas Merton* (pp. 29-42). Notre Dame, IN: Ave Maria Press.
Epictetus. (1968). Encheiridion. In Walter Kaufman (Ed.), *Philosophic classics: Thales to Ockham* (pp. 477-490). Hoboken, NJ: Prentice Hall.
Flaxman, G. (2012). *Gilles Deleuze and the fabulation of philosophy*. Minneapolis, MN: University of Minnesota Press.
Foucault, M. (1969). *The archaeology of knowledge*. France: Editions Gallimard.
Foucault, M. (1988). *Madness and civilization: A history of insanity in the age of reason*. New York: Vintage.
Foucault, M. (1994a). *The birth of the clinic: An archaeology of medical perception*. New York: Vintage.
Foucault, M. (1994b). *The order of things: An archaeology of the human sciences*. New York: Vintage.
Foucault, M. (1995). *Discipline and punish: The birth of the prison*. New York: Vintage.
Foucault, M. (2008a). *The birth of biopolitics: Lectures at the College de France, 1978-1979* (Transl., Graham Burchell). New York: Palgrave Macmillan.
Foucault, M. (2010). *The government of self and others: Lectures at the college de France, 1982-1983* (Transl., Graham Burchell). New York: Palgrave Macmillan.
Foucault, M. (2011). *The courage of truth: Lectures at the college de France, 1983-1984*. New York: Palgrave.
Frank, A. (1997). *The wounded storyteller: Body, illness, and ethics*. Chicago: University of Chicago Press.
Freud, S. (1917). *Mourning and melancholia*. SE (Transl., James Strachey). New York: W. W. Norton.
Freud, S. (1953). *A case of hysteria: Three essays on sexuality and other works*. Standard Edition (SE) (Transl., James Strachey). Londong: The Hogarth Press.
Freud, S. (1989). *Civilizations and its discontents*. SE (Transl., James Strachey). New York: W.W. Norton.

Freud, S. (1993). *Three case histories: The "wolf man," the "rat man," and the psychotic doctor Schreber.* Philip Rieff (Ed.). New York: Simon & Schuster.
Fynsk, C. (1991). Foreword. Experiences of finitude. In, Jean-Luc Nancy, *The inoperative community* (pp. vii–xxxv). Minneapolis, MN: The University of Minnesota Press.
Gleick, J. (1987). *Chaos: Making a new science.* New York: Penguin.
Gramsci, A. (1971). *Selections from the prison notebooks* (Transl., Quintin Hoare & Geoffrey Nowell Smith). New York: International Publishers.
Gramsci, A. (2000). *The Antonio Gramsci Reader: Selected writings 1916-1935.* David Forgacs (Ed.). New York: New York University Press.
Grayling, A. C. (2019). *The history of philosophy.* New York: Penguin.Green, A. (1993). *Private madness.* Madison, CT: International Universities Press.
Gregg, R. (1980). Introduction. In, *Athanasius the life of Antony and the letter to Marcellinus* (pp. 1-26). Mahwah, NJ: Paulist Press.
Gubar, S. (2012). *Memoir of a debulked woman: Enduring ovarian cancer.* New York: W. W. Norton.
Gunther, J. (1949). *Death be not proud.* New York: Harper Perrennial.
Haraway, D. (1997). *Modest_witness@second_millennium. Femaleman_meets_oncomouse: Feminism and Technoscience.* New York: Routledge.
Haraway, D. (2011). *Donna Haraway SF: Speculative fabulation on string figures.* Vol. 33. Germany: Hatje Cantz Verlag.
Harmless, W. (2004). *Desert Christians: An introduction to the literature of monasticism.* New York: Oxford.
Hegel, G. F. W. (1977). *Phenomenology of spirit* (Transl., A.V. Miller). New York: Oxford University Press.
Heidegger, M. (1926/1962). *Being and time* (Transl., John Macquarrie & Edward Robinson). New York: Harper & Row Publishers.
Heidegger, M. (2017a). *Ponderings II-VI: Black notebooks, 1931-1938* (Transl., Richard Rojcewicz). Bloomington, IN: Indiana University Press.
Heidegger, M. (2017b). *Ponderings VII-XI: Black notebooks, 1938-1939* (Transl., Richard Rojcewicz). Bloomington, IN: Indiana University Press.
Heidegger, M. (2017c). *Ponderings XII-XV: Black notebooks, 1939-1941* (Transl., Richard Rojcewicz). Bloomington, IN: Indiana University Press.
Hesse, H. (1943/1990). *The glass bead game.* New York: Picador. Henry Hold & Company.
Hillman, J. (1975). *Loose ends: primary papers in archetypal psychology.* Putnam, CT: Spring Publications.
Hillman, J. (1983). *Healing fiction.* Putnam, CT: Spring Publications.
Huebner, D. (1999). *The lure of the transcendent: Collected essays by Dwayne E. Huebner.* Vikki Hillis (Ed.) Collected and introduced by William F. Pinar. Mahwah, NJ: Lawrence Erlbaum and Associates Publishers.
James, W. (1958). *The varieties of religious experience.* New York: The New American Library.
James, W. (2000). *Pragmatism and other writings.* New York: Penguin.
Jauhar, S. (2008). *Intern: A doctor's initiation.* New York: Farrar, Straus and Giroux.
Jay, M. (2020). *Splinters in your eye: Frankfurt school provocations.* New York: Verso.

Jenkyns, R. (2007). Introduction. In, Lucretius, *The nature of things* (pp. vii–xxiii). New York: Penguin.
Jensen, D. (2000). *A language older than words.* New York: Context Books.
Kafka, F. (1915). *Gatekeeper before the law.* Prague: Czechoslovakia: *Selbstwehr.*
Kant, I. (1979). *The conflict of the faculties* (Transl., Mary J. Gregor). New York: Abaris.
Kant, I. (2002). *Critique of practical reason.* Indianapolis, IN: Hackett Publishing.
Kant, I. (2007). *Critique of pure reason.* New York: Penguin.
Kaufman, W. (1968). *Philosophic classics volume 1: Thales to Ockham.* Englewood Cliffs, NJ: Prentice Hall.
Keller, R. C. (2007). *Colonial madness: Psychiatry in French North Africa.* Chicago: The University of Chicago Press. Kierkegaard, S. (1973; 1854-1855). The attack upon "Christendom" *(1954-1855).* In Robert Bretall (Ed.), *A Kierkegaard anthology* (pp. 434-468). Princeton, NJ: Princeton University Press.
Kierkegaard, S. (1983). *Fear and trembling: Repetition* (Transl., Howard V. Hong & Edna H. Hong). NJ: Princeton University Press.
Kierkegaard, S. (1987). *Either/or. Volume 1* (Transl., Howard V. Hong & Edna H. Hong). Princeton, NJ: Princeton University Press.
Kierkegaard, S. (1988). *Stages on life's way* (Transl., Howard V. Hong & Edna H. Hong). Princeton, NJ: Princeton University Press.
Klein, M. (1992). *Love, guilt and reparation and other works, 1921-1945.* London: Karnac.
Klein, M. (1993). *Envy and gratitude and other works, 1946-1963.* London: Karnac.
Langer, S. (1957). *Philosophy in a new key: A study in the symbolism of reason, rite, and art.* Cambridge, MA: Harvard University Press.
Leeming, D. A. (2014). *The world of myth: An anthology.* New York: Oxford University Press.
Leibniz, G.W. (2020). *Discourse on metaphysics* (Transl., Gonzalo Rodriguez-Pereyra). Oxford, UK: Oxford University Press.
Levinas, E. (1985). *Ethics and infinity* (Transl., Richard A. Cohen). Pittsburgh, PA: Duquesne University Press.
Levinas, E. (1996). *Basic philosophical writings*Adriaan. T. Peperzak, Simon Critchley & Robert Bernasconi (Eds.). Bloomington, IN: Indiana University Press.
Levinas, E. (2000). *God, death, and time.* Stanford, CA: Stanford University Press.
Lorcin, P. (2014). Politics, artistic merit, and the posthumous reputation of Albert Camus. *The South Central Review* (Vol. 33), No. 3, pp. 9-26.
Lottman, H. R. (1997). *Albert Camus: A Biography.* Corte Madera, CA: Gingko Press.
Lucretius. (2007). *The nature of things* (Transl., A. E. Stallings). New York: Penguin.
Luria, A. R. (1968). *The mind of a mnemonist: A little book about a vast memory* (Transl., Lynn Solotaroff). Cambridge, MA: Harvard University Press.
Luria, A. R. (2002). *The man with a shattered world: The history of a brain wound* (Transl., Lynn Solotaroff). Cambridge, MA: Harvard University Press.
Macdonald, J. (1995). *Curriculum as a prayerful act.* New York: Peter Lang.
Malabou, C. (2008). *What should we do with our brain?* (Transl., Sebastian Rand). New York: Fordham University Press.

Marcel, G. (1950). *The mystery of being, Volume II: Faith and reality* (Transl., G.S. Fraser). South Bend, IN: St. Augustine's Press.

Marno, D. (2016). *Death be not proud: The art of holy attention.* Chicago: University of Chicago Press.

Marty, E. (2018). A throw of the dice by Stephen Mallarme. In *Diptyqueparis-memento.com.* September 17.

Marx, K. (1967). Economic and philosophic manuscripts (1844). In *Writings of the Young Marx on philosophy and society* (Eds. & Transl., Loyd D. Easton & Kurt H. Guddat) (pp. 283-318). New York: Doubleday.

Mattiessen, P. (1978). *The snow leopard.* New York: Viking.

Mayers, G. (2014). *Listen to the desert: Secrets of spiritual maturity from the desert fathers and mothers.* Chicago: Acta Publications.

Mbembe, A. (2019). *Necropolitics.* Durhram, NC: Duke University Press.

Merleau-Ponty, M. (1968). *The visible and the invisible* (Transl., Alphonso Lingis). Evanston, IL: Northwestern University Press.

Merleau-Ponty, M. (1989). *The primacy of perception.* Evanston, IL: Northwestern University Press.

Merleau-Ponty, M. (2010). *Phenomenology of perception.* New York: Routledge.

Merton, T. (1955). *No man is an island.* New York: A Harvest Book.

Merton, T. (1960). *The wisdom of the desert.* New York: New Directions.

Merton, T. (1966). *Raids on the unspeakable.* New York: New Directions.

Merton, T. (1972). *New seeds of contemplation.* New York: New Directions.

Merton, T. (1981). *The ascent to truth.* New York: A Harvest Book.

Merton, T. (1998). *The seven storey mountain: An autobiography of faith.* New York: A Harvest Book.

Merton, T. (2007a). *Echoing silence: Thomas Merton on the vocation of writing.* Boston: New Seeds Publishing.

Merton, T. (2007b). *Thomas Merton: A book of hours.* Notre Dame, IN: Sorin Books.

Merton, T. (2019). *A course in desert spirituality.* Collegeville, Minnesota: Liturgical Press.

Miller, A. (2001). *The truth will set you free: Overcoming emotional blindness and finding your true adult self.* New York: Basic Books.

Morris, M. (2001). *Curriculum and the Holocaust: Competing sites of memory and representation.* New York: Routledge.

Morris, M. (2008). *Teaching through the ill body: A spiritual and aesthetic approach to pedagogy and illness* (Educational philosophy and theory, Vol. 54, 2022-Issue 4). Rotterdam, The Netherlands: Sense Publishers.

Morris, M. (2016a; 2016b). *Curriculum studies guidebooks: Concepts and Theoretical Frameworks.* New York: Peter Lang.

Morris, M. (2021a). *Chaplaincy during the age of covid-19.* Column in PESA AGORA: A meeting place of ideas. *pesaagora.com.*

Morris, M. (2021b). Michel Serres: Divergences. In *Educational philosophy and theory,* May. Sense Publishers.

Musil, R. (1996a). *The man without qualities. Vol. 1.* New York: Vintage.

Musil, R. (1996b). *The man without qualities. Vol. 2.* New York: Vintage.

Nancy, J-L. (1991). *The inoperative community* (Transl., Peter Conner, Lisa Garbus, Michael Holland & Simona Sawhney). Minneapolis, MN: University of Minnesota Press.

Nancy, J-L. (1996). *The muses* (Transl., Peggy Kamuf). Stanford, CA: Stanford University Press.

Nancy, J.-L. (1997). *The sense of the world* (Transl., Jeffrey S. Librett). Minneapolis, MN: University of Minnesota Press.

Newman, J. H. (1852). *The idea of a university defined and illustrated: Discourses delivered to the Catholics of Dublin.* London: Longman's, Green & Company.

Nietzsche, F. (1974). *The gay science* (Transl., Walter Kaufman). New York: Vintage.

Nietzsche, F. (1989). *Beyond good and evil: Prelude to a philosophy of the future* (Transl., Walter Kaufman). New York: Vintage.

Nietzsche, F. (1997). *Daybreak: Thoughts on the prejudices of morality* (Transl., R. J. Hollingdale). Cambridge, UK: Cambridge University Press.

Nietzsche, F. (2000). On the genealogy of morals. In Walter Kaufman (Ed.), *Basic writings of Nietzsche* (pp. 437-600). New York: The Modern Library.

Nietzsche, F. (2004). *On the future of our educational institutions.* South Bend, IN: St. Augustine's Press.

Nietzsche, F. (2008). *Twilight of idols* (Transl., Duncan Large). New York: Oxford University Press.

Nietzsche, F. (2009). *Ecce homo* (Transl., Duncan Large). New York: Oxford University Press.

Nietzsche, F. (2010). *The anti-Christ.* Columbia, SC: SoHo Books.

Nietzsche, F. (2017). *The will to power.* New York: Penguin.

Nowen, H. (2010). *The wounded healer: Ministry in contemporary society.* New York: Doubleday.

Oransky, I. (2014). "Nobel prize winner calls peer review "very distorted," "completely corrupt," and "simply a regression to the mean." (*Retractionwatch.com*, March 2, 2014).

Parmenides. (1984). In David Gallop (Ed. & Transl.), *Parmenides of Elea: Fragments.* Toronto, Canada: University of Toronto Press.

Peeters, B. (2013). *Derrida: A biography.* Malden, MA: Polity.

Peirce, C. S. (1877). The fixation of belief. *Popular science Monthly*, 12, November, pp. 1-15.

Peirce, C. S. (1955). The doctrine of necessity examined. In Justus Buchler (Ed.), *Philosophical Writings of C. S. Peirce* (pp. 324-338). New York: Dover Publications, Inc.

Phillips, A. (2001). *Houdini's box: The art of escape.* New York: Pantheon.

Phillips, A. (2012). *Missing out: In praise of the unlived life.* New York: Farrar, Straus and Giroux.

Pike, B. (1996). Translator's afterword. In Robert Musil's *Man without qualities. Vol. 11* (pp. 1771-1774). New York: Vintage.

Pinar, W. F., et al. (1995). *Understanding curriculum.* New York: Peter Lang.

Pinar, W. F. (2009). *The worldliness of a cosmopolitan education: Passionate lives in public service.* New York: Routledge.

Plato (2008a). The apology. In, *Plato: The Complete works of Plato, volume II* (Transl, Benjamin Jowett) (pp. 61-76). London, UK: Akasha Publishing Ltd.

Plato (2008b). The timaeus. In, *Plato: The Complete works of Plato, Volume II* (Transl., Benjamin Jowett) (pp. 645-689). London, UK: Akasha Publishing Ltd.

Plato (2012). *The Republic* (Transl., Benjamin Jowett). New York: Penguin.

Popper, K. R. (1990). *A world of propensities.* Bristol: Thoemmes Antiquarian Book, Ltd.

Rahner, K. (1992). *Karl Rahner: Theologian of theologian of the graced search for meaning.* Minneapolis, MN: Fortress Press.

Reck, A. J. (1972). *Speculative philosophy: A study of its nature, types and uses.* Albuquerque, NM: University of New Mexico Press.

Ricoeur, P. (1970). *Freud and philosophy: An essay on interpretation.* New Haven, CT: Yale University Press.

Rokeach, M. (1964/2011). *The three Christs of Ypsilanti.* New York: NYRB.

Ronell, A. (2002). *Stupidity.* Urbana, IL: University of Illinois Press.

Royce, J. (2001). *The problem of Christianity.* Washington DC: The Catholic University Press of America.

Russell, B. (1957). *Why I am not a Christian and other essays and related subjects.* New York: Simon & Schuster.

Sacks, O. (1990). *Awakenings.* New York: Vintage.

Sacks, O. (1998). *The man who mistook his wife for a hat and other clinical tales.* New York: Simon & Schuster.

Sacks, O. (2010). *The mind's eye.* New York: Random House.

Said, E. W. (1979). *Orientalism.* New York: Vintage.

Said, E. W. (1996). *Representations of the intellectual.* New York: Vintage.

Salmon, P. (2020). *An event, perhaps: A biography of Jacques Derrida.* New York: Verso.

Salvio, P. (2017). *The story-takers: Public pedagogy, transitional justice, and Italy's non-violent protest against the Mafia.* Toronto: The University of Toronto Press.

Sartre, J-P. (1961). Preface. In, Frantz Fanon, *Wretched of the earth* (pp. xliii–xlxii). New York: Vintage.

Schnabel, J. (2018). *At eternity's gate.* Director Julian Schnabel. Riverstone Pictures.

Schrader, P. (2018). *First reformed.* Director Paul Schrader. A24 Films.

Schreber, D. P. (2000). *Memoirs of my nervous illness.* New York: NYRB Classics.

Seneca. (2018). *How to die: An ancient guide to the end of life* (Transl., James S. Romm). Princeton, NJ: Princeton University Press.

Serres, M. (1983). *Hermes: Literature, science, philosophy.* Baltimore, MD: The Johns Hopkins University Press.

Serres, M. (1991). *Rome: Book of foundations* (Transl., Felicia McCarren). Stanford, CA: Stanford University Press.

Serres, M. (1993). *Angels: A modern myth.* Paris, France: Flammarion.

Serres, M. (1995). *Genesis* (Transl., Genevieve James & James Nielson). Ann Arbor, MI: University of Michigan Press.

Serres, M. (1998). *Serres/Latour. Michel Serres with Bruno Latour: Conversations on science, culture, and time* (Transl., Roxanne Lapidus). Ann Arbor, MI: The University of Michigan Press.

Serres, M. (2001). *The birth of physics* (Transl., David Webb & William Ross). New York: Rowman & Littlefield.

Serres, M. (2007). *The parasite* (Transl., Lawrence Schehr). Minneapolis, MN: Minnesota University Press.

Serres, M. (2012). *Biogea* (Transl., Randolph Burks). Minneapolis, MN: Univocal Publishing.

Skloot, R. (2011). *The immortal life of Henrietta Lacks.* New York: Crown.

St. John (2017). *The collected works of St. John of the cross* (Transl., Kieran Kavanaugh & Otilio Rodrigeuz). Washington, DC: ICS Publications. Institute of Carmelite Studies.

Stone, P. (2016). Russell the political activist. In Tim Madigan & Peter Stone (Eds.), *Bertrand Russell: Public intellectual* (pp. 99-132). Rochester, NY: Tiger Bark Press.

Taylor, C. C. W. (2010). *The atomists: Leucippus and Democritus* (Transl., C. C. W. Taylor). Toronto: University of Toronto Press.

Thoreau, H. D. (2021). *Walden with the duty of civil disobedience.* New York: Reader's Library Classic.

Tillich, P. (1970). *Ultimate concern.* New York: HarperCollins.

Todd, O. (2000). *Albert Camus: A life* (Transl., Benjamin Ivry). New York: Carroll & Graf Publishers, Inc.

Tucker, R. C. (1978). Introduction. In, *The Marx-Engels Reader* (pp. xix–xlii). New York: W. W. Norton.

Turley, H., Martin, D. (2018). *The martyrdom of Thomas Merton: An investigation.* Scotts Valley, CA: CreateSpace Independent Platform.

Tyler, R. W. (1969). *Basic principles of curriculum and instruction.* Chicago: University of Chicago Press.

Young, I. (1977). *Heidegger, philosophy, Nazism.* New York: Cambridge University Press.

Urrea, L. A. (2004). *The Devil's highway.* New York: Back Bay Books.

Viallaneix, P. (1977). The First Camus. In *Youthful writings: Albert Camus* (pp. 3-103). New York: Vintage.

Von Umwerth, M. (2005). *Freud's requiem: Mourning, melancholia and the invisible history of a summer walk.* New York: Riverhead Books/Penguin.

Vulor, E. C. (2000). *Colonial and anti-colonial discourses: Albert Camus and Algeria.* Lanham, MD University Press of America.

Weatherhill, R. (1998). *The sovereignty of death.* London: Rebus Press.

Ward, B. (1975). *The sayings of the desert fathers: The alphabetic collection.* Collegeville, MN: Cistercian Publications.

Whitehead, A. N. (1927). *Process and reality: An essay in cosmology. Gifford Lectures.* New York: The Free Press.

Whitehead, A. N. (1929). *The aims of education and other essays.* New York: The Free Press.

Williams, T. T. (2001). *Refuge: An unnatural history of family and place.* New York: Vintage.

Winnicott, D. W. (2005). *Playing and reality.* New York: Routledge.

Wittgenstein, L. (1922). *The tractatus logico-philosophicus* (Transl., Frank R. Ramsey). New York: Kegan Paul.

Wittgenstein, L. (1958). *Philosophical investigations* (Transl., G.E. M. Anscombe). Saddle River, NJ: Prentice Hall.

Zaretsky, R. (2010). *Albert Camus: Elements of a life.* Ithaca, NY: Cornell University Press.

Zizek, S. (2020). *Hegel in a wired brain.* New York: Bloomsbury Academic.

Index

A

abandonment, 118, 167
Abraham, Nicholas, 165
Abram, David, 67
abstractions, 175
abstract philosopher, 175–6
academic freedom, 103
Adieu: To Emmanuel Levinas, 205
administered world, 38
administrators, 39, 77, 104
administrivia, 101
Agathon, 16
ageism, 37
Agora, 152
AIDS, 179
Alice in *Wonderland*, 50
alterity
    archiving, 68–9
    concept, 66–8
    decimated, 66
    description, 66
Anachoresis-solitude, 22
Angels: A Modern Myth, 202
Angelus Novaus, 56
anthropologists, 41
anticipation, 73, 74
Anti-Oedipus, 132
anti-Semitism, 96, 178, 185, 186
Antony, 13
Anzaldua, Gloria, 82
apocalyptic literature, 9
apolitical ideology, 153
Apology, 49, 176
aporia, 118
Arcades Project, 75
arche-phenomenon of memory, 120
architectonic organization, 142
archivization, 71–4
    context, 74
    différance, 80–3
    ethical obligation, 84
    historiography, 72, 75

218 | Index

is historicity, 86
Messianic time, 73
movement, 173
Arendt, Hannah, 55, 134, 142, 143, 152, 192
Aristotle, 49, 50
Arius (Libyan theologian), 11, 12
asceticism, 22
Athanasius, 15
Attacks upon Christendom, 92
authentic relationship, 65, 67
authoritarianism, 180
autobiography, 4
aversion to death, 3

B

Bachelard, Gaston, 16, 50
Badiou, Alain, 121, 193
Balibar, Etienne, 81
ball-games, 61
Baptism, 29
Barnes, Julian, 80
Before the Law, 39
Being and Time, 143
Benjamin, Walter, 47, 48, 53–7, 72, 74, 101, 102, 121, 174
Bergson, Henri, 47, 52, 128
Berlin Chronicle, 53
Beyond Good and Evil, 191
Biblical scholars, 9
bioethicists, 43
biogeochemistry, 52
The Birth of Physics, 188, 194
The Birth of the Clinic, 25, 31
Black Notebooks, 143, 144
Blanchot, Maurice, 201
blank place, 198
board-games, 61
body-bags, 6

Boisen, Anton, 206
dissociation of doctor and patient, 142
emotional distress, 144
experience with doctor, 142
Freudian psychoanalysis, 142
hospital chaplaincy, 142
memoir, 139
mental problems, 145
psyche, 141
psychiatric patients, 141
speculation, 142
students of chaplaincy, 140
Bollas, Christopher, 169
Bonhoeffer, Dietrich, 73, 99, 106
Bree, Germaine, 170, 182
Brenner, Sydney, 53
Bubonic Plague in Europe, 44
Buddhist literature, 66
bureaucracy of administration, 77
Butler, Judith, 32, 38, 145, 159, 202, 206

C

CA-125, 32
"Call it", 36
Camus, Albert, 10, 206
biography, 178
critiques, 183–6
Father Paneloux, 178–80
longings and temptations, 161
philosophers, 162–72
self-education, 182–3
cancer, 3
context of, 158
ovarian, 6
patients, 158
card-games, 61
Carol, Lewis, 50
Carretto, Carlo, 7, 22
Carson, Rachel, 118
Cartesian scientific method, 83

Casey, Edward, 18
Cassier, Ernst, 98
catastrophic archivization, 69–71
Catholic theology, 92
chaos narrative, 41
chaos theorists, 194
chaplains, 169, 202
    charts (see charts)
    empirical observation, 32
    medical model, 31
    narratives, 29–30, 34
    verbatim conversations, 31, 34
chaplaincy program, 5, 59
Charity, 22
chart notes, 43
charts
    basic formula, 33
    check a box, 29–31
    checklists, 29
    computerized databases, 29
    configurations, 36
    description, 30
    medical, 29
    notes, 43
    physicians, 29
    spiritual outcome, 29
cheap pleasure, 19
check a box, charts, 29–31
chemotherapy, 159
Chomsky, Noam, 152
Christendom, 73
Christian anti-Semitism, 178
Christianity, 92
Christian scriptures, 9
Christian theology, 11
Christocentrism, 73
Christology, 11–15
chronicles, 48, 53–4
Chryssavgis, John, 8, 21
cinders, 74
Cistercian Order, 14
classism, 37

clergy, 12
clinical case studies, 37–40, 43
Clinical Pastoral Education (CPE), 5
Clock-Time, 2
code alteration mutates things, 52
code blues, 203
coffeehouses, 101
College of Pastoral Supervision and
    Psychotherapy (CPSP)
    chaplaincy programs, 5
    hospital administrators, 5
    religion, 5
    standardized clinical narratives, 5
color blindness, 133
common-sense thinking, 33
commons-of-covid, 89
Communism, 185
Communist Manifesto, 185–6
conceptualization, 86
confessions, 14, 97, 100
configurations, 36
Conflict of the Faculties, 105
conservative legislators, 114
conspirator, 47
contemplation
    and action, 97–8
contingency, 189
continual catastrophe, 90
corpses, 37
cosmology, 188
cosmos, 196
The Cost of Discipleship, 106
The Courage of Truth, 42, 153
courage of truth (book), 86
    authoritarianism(s), 96
    crisis, 95
    false hope, 94
    false piety, 93
    negative truth, 93
    pretending, 93
    work of mourning, 95
covid-19, 5

catastrophes, 44
child who loses parent, 94
collision of, 159
deaths, 6, 159
delta variant, 35
Derrida's concepts, 84–7
emergence of, 41
families, 30–1
fight for the oppressed past, 55
hospitals, 24
life catastrophes, 24
medical staff, 125
other's death, 124
pandemic, 4
patients and death, 125
patients, 35, 115
refrigerator storage, 125
speculative fabulation, 63
treatments, 37
unvaccinated, 193
vaccinated, 123
violence, 195
wards, 115
covid kills, 87
covid pandemic, 172–5
crisis of *parrhesia*, 155
cross-disciplinary
  fashion, 196
  studies, 196
crystal-clear blue sea, 170
cultural collision, 43
Currere, 140, 173
  aversion, 3
  ecological concept, 3
  eco-theological crisis, 3
  socio-political, 3
curriculum, 85
  studies, 6
  theory, 97
Cynic-as-spy, 48
Cynics, 176

D

Dadedalus, 50–1
death, 10, 74, 203
  "complicated", 116
  inhumane, 125
  occurrence, 121
  during pandemic, 109
  "quick", 116
  refrigerator storage, 125
Death Be Not Proud, 18, 157
deaths
  bodies, refrigerated drawers, 36
  covid-19, 35
  morgue, 36
  plastic bags, 36
decimated alterity, 66
deconstruction, 82, 83, 101
Deignan, Kathleen, 106
DeLancey, Craig, 185
Deleuze, Gilles, 71
deliberation, 76
deltacron variants, 158
delta variant, 158
delusions, 141
Democritus, 192
demons, 15
depression, 141, 167
De Rerum Nartura, 187
Derrida (film), 162
Derrida, Jacques, 25, 105, 109, 161, 162
  abandoned archive, 70
  alterity, 68–9
  archeology, 70
  archivization, 68–9, 75
  border-conflicts, 105
  covid, 109
  differance, 80–3
  Freudian archivization, 69
  Freudian project, 70
  Lacanian psychoanalysis, 70
  Messianism, 54

pandemic, 84–7
philosophy, 75
profanely-sacred sense, 70
reader's interpretation, 161
speculative fabulation, 25
trace, 74–80
trace and difference, 65
transcencendence, 72
university-to-come, 77
Derrida: A Biography, 177
DeSalvo, Louise, 168, 206
   childhood trauma, 148
   family members, 149
   The House of Early Sorrows, 148
   ICU beds, 151
   incest, 148
   memoirs, 149
   memory traces, 149
   self-hatred and violence, 149
Descartes's *Meditations,* 20
desert-like madness, 15
despondency, 17
destruction, 167
Devereux, George, 162
Diat, Nicolas, 21, 115–16
Didion, Joan, 58, 206
   covid, 128
   disbeliefs, 131
   forever-ness of death, 127
   grief, 127
   husband's death, 127, 128, 130
   magical thinking, 126, 128–31
   memoir, 127
   philosophy, 129–30
   rage, 131
   unbearable story, 129
   Year of Magical Thinking, 126
différance, 80–3
différance-as-allegory, 81
Diogenes, 181
Discipline and Punish (book), 42
documentation, 36
Doll, Mary, 2

Donne, John, 18
drug seeking, 38
duck-rabbit, 60, 61
   puzzle, 133
duty and responsibility, 5

E

Ecce Homo, 202
Echographies, 82
Echographies of Television, 76
Echoing Silence, 102
ecology of death, 17–20
economy of words, 20–2
Educare, 49
Ellsberg, Robert, 13
emergency rooms, 30
   chaos and confusion, 32
emotional exhaustion, 35
empathy, 204
Empedocles, 17, 195–6, 205
empiricism, 58, 98
encephalitis lethargica, 45
Enlightenment, 142, 144, 145
   philosophy, 96
Epicurus, 120, 121, 123, 187, 189, 194
epidemiologists, 201
ethical work, 73
The Ethics, 49
Eudamonia, 50
An Event, Perhaps: A Biography of Jacques Derrida, 177
ever-moving process, 5
evildoers, 179
The Exploration of the Inner World, 26
extubation, 201

F

fabulations, 25, 48, 51
   perception, 62
   speculation, 62
Face of God, 72
Facts and Fable in Psychology, 60
faculty members, 104
Fadiman, Anne, 41, 43
false negatives, 200
family violence, 137
Fanon, Frantz, 184
fascism, 153
Father Paneloux, 178–80, 190
felt-as-memory, 47
Ferlinghetti, Lawrence, 102
fictional multiple integral equation, 52
figure in the carpet, 57
first-hand witness, 24
The First Man, 26, 163–5, 177, 183
first meditation, metaphors of the desert
   madness, 15
   myth, madness and archetypes, 16
   the sublime, 9–10
   theology, 11
   thoughts of death, 7–9
Fixation of Belief, 19
fixed beliefs, 20
flashes, 54
Flaxman, Gregory, 48
flight of the unattainable, 51
flights after the unattainable, 57
floods, 194
1918 flu pandemic, 44, 56, 200
for-profit hospitals, 34, 147
Foucault, Michel, 25, 31, 42, 48, 142, 176
Fox, Matthew, 91, 92
frame of reference, 33
Francis of Assisi, Saint, 146
Frank, Arthur, 41

freedom, 56
French-Algerian War, 167
frustration, 151
future-of-no-future, 84
Fynsk, Christopher, 79, 85

G

gatekeepers, 104
Genesis, 195
germ atom, 200
ghosts, 159
Ginsburg, Allen, 102
Gleick, James, 189, 198
global scale, 113
global warming, 132, 136, 194
gloss over, 54
god, 50, 90, 191–2
   existence, 90
Goffman, Erving, 102
Gough, Van, 51
Gramsci, Antonio, 100
Grass, Gunter, 185
Great Salt Lake, 2
Greek philosophers, 42
Green, Andre, 165, 171, 172
Gregory of Nyssa, St., 97
grief, compounded, 2
Guattari, Felix, 71
Gubar, Susan, 158
guilt, 167
Gunther, John, 26, 206
   courageous struggle, 157
   Greek philosophers, 156
   gut-wrenching story, 154
   memoir, 155, 159
   negation, 157
   physicians, 155
   radical relativism, 155
   son's death, 154
   truth-tellers, 155–6

gun violence, 109

H

hallucinations, 10–11, 141
Haraway, Donna, 25, 48, 52, 196
Harmless, William, 12
health care professionals, 151
health humanities, 40
Hebbs, Donald, 98
Hebrew scriptures, 9
Hegel Spirit, 143
Heidegger, Martin, 52
Hermes: Literature, Science, Philosophy, 193
Hesse, Herman, 107
Hillman, James, 30, 33, 58
historical constellation, 72
historicity-as-archivization, 86
Historiography, 48
Hitler's Final Solution, 104
Holocaust, 66, 115
Holocaust deniers, 55
homogeneous empty time, 47, 48, 54–5
"homogeneous" experience, 128
Homoousious, 11
Homo Sapiens, 52
hospital chaplains, 6, 9, 19, 114
hospital chaplaincy, 139, 147
The House of Early Sorrows, 26, 148
houses bureaucracies, 103
Huebner, Dwayne, 6, 98
humanities, 34, 103, 147
hysteria, 120

I

Icarus, Greek myth, 50–1
The Idea of the University, 106

implosion, 197
inconvenient truths, 136
inflation, 151
inner discipline, 20
The Inoperative Community, 108
inscription, 110
intellectual freedom, 105, 106
intellectualism, 122, 143
intellectual virtue, 49
interference, 197
interpretation, 86
intersubjectivity, 59
intubation, 201
islamophobia, 184

J

James, Henry, 57
James, William, 58, 139, 140, 146
Jauhar, Sandeep, 18, 19
Jay, Martin, 136
Jenkyns, Richard, 187, 194
Jensen, Derrick, 150, 168
  cultural violence, 135, 136
  culture, 135
  devastation, 132
  ecological activist, 132
  family violence, 137
  father, abusive, 132–4
  gaslighting, 134
  life project, 136
  perception, 133
  Prussian system, 135
  refuge in nature, 132
  unbearable stories, 137
Jesus the Christ, 11–12
Jesus' visions, 15
John of the Cross, St., 93–4, 96
Joshua Tree, 3
The Joshua Tree (album), 1
The Joshua Tree National Park, 1

The Jungle, 149

K

Kaufman, Walter, 176
Keller, Richard, 185
Kierkegaard, Soren, 92
Klee, Paul, 55, 56
Klein, Melanie, 166, 167

L

Langer, Sussanne, 98
language-games, 61
lax policies, 5
L-Dopa drug, 44–5
Lemming, David, 50
Levinas, Emmanuel, 65
　alterity concept, 66–8
Leviticus (book), 8
Lewis, Sinclair, 135
liberation theology, 99
liberty, 56
Life changes in the instant, 129
life never lived, 56–9
lightning, 194
Logomachia: The Conflict of the Faculties, 103
Lorcin, Patricia, 185
Lottman, Herbert, 165
Lucretius, 120, 121, 123, 187–9
The Lure of the Transcendent, 98
Luria, A.R., 25, 39
Luther, Martin, 92

M

Macdonald, James, 6, 97

Magic Mountain (novel), 183
Mann, Thomas, 183
The Man with A Shattered World (2002), 39
The Man Without Qualities, 96, 178
The Man with the Shattered World, 25
Marcel, Gabriel, 89, 90
Margins of Philosophy, 76
Marin, Louis, 205
Marshall, John, 23
Martin, David, 98
Marxism, 112
Matthiessen, Peter, 67
McDonaldization, 34, 36
Mead, George Herbert, 153
medical anthropologists, 43
medical anthropology, 41–2
medical chart, 29
medical community, 38, 43
medical humanities, 40, 147
medical materialism, 140, 141
medical professionals, 159
Mediocrity, 53
The *Meditations,* 20
melancholia, 64
melancholy, 54
Memoirists, 173
Memoir of My Nervous Illness, 15
Memorial University Medical Center Hospital in Savannah, 5
memory, 73
mental life, 56
Merleau-Ponty, Maurice, 59–60, 97, 130
Merton, Thomas, 2, 8, 10–12, 14, 59, 137, 206
　activist and writer, 91
　autobiography, 100
　contemplation and action, 97–8
　courage of truth, 93–7
　death, 99
　pessimism, 91

philosopher-poet, 102
and political engagement, 98–110
realistic theologians, 90
theology, 89
Trappist Monk, 91
unspeakable crisis (see unspeakable)
Messianic time, 59, 72, 73
Messianism, 54, 83
metanarratives, 75
metaphors of the desert
biography, 4
covid-19, 4
flu epidemic, 4
horror and tragedy, 4
intersection of, 5
madness, 15
mirages/hallucinations, 10–11
myth, madness and archetypes, 16
the sublime, 9–10
theology, 11
thoughts of death, 7–9
Metaphysical quandaries, 51
metaphysics, 75, 76
Miller, Alice, 150
The Mind of a Mnemonist (1968), 39, 40
The Mind's Eye, 133
mirages, 10–11
mirror-of-the-mind, 10
misogyny, 119
mobs, 15
monastic life rule, 13
Moore, Thomas, 58
moral action, 50
moral virtue, 49
mortality, 64
mourning, 64
multiplicity, 52
multi-substance, 38
Musil, Robert, 96, 178
My Nervous Illness, 132
the mystical writing pad, 78
myth, madness and archetypes, 16

The Myth of Sisyphus, 168, 169, 171

N

Nancy, Jean-Luc, 108–10, 203
narratives, 42–5
necropolitics, 37, 151
negative truth, 93
neo-liberal university, 147
Neo-Nazism, 96
neurological problems, 45
Newman, John Henry, 106
Nicaean Creed, 11
The Nichomachean Ethics, 49, 158
"no frame of reference", 33
noise, 195–7
The Noise of Time, 80
noncompliant, 38
non-conceptual, 85
nonconceptualities, 112, 121
non-for-profit hospitals, 34
non-human animal, 67
no-nonsense legal documents, 34
non-symmetrical, 67
normality is death, 55
not-looking-forward, 67
Nouwen, Henri, 21

O

omicron, 111, 158
Oregon, 194
Orff, Carl, 80
organic difficulty, 140
originative principle, 23
The Origins of Totalitarianism, 180
Orthodoxy, 11–15
Otto, Rudolph, 3
ovarian cancers, 6, 32, 119, 120

over-generalizations, 38

P

Painting, 51
Palm Springs, 1
  in California, 1
  Joshua Tree National Park, 2
  New Year's Celebration, 2
Palm trees, 2
pandemic
  covid patients, 35
  death and trauma, 35
  emotional exhaustion, 35
  ever-changing, 199
  fluid relationship, 199
  historians, 199
  metaphors, 198
  television, 202
  unvaccinated, 200
pandemic rages, 151
pandemonium, 115, 199
Paneloux, 178–80
paradigm shifts, 42
paradoxical nature, 71–4
paranoia, 167
paranoid-schizophrenics, 167
paraphrasing, 68, 79
parents, 195
Parkinsonian-like symptoms, 45
Parmenides, 120, 174–5, 192
parrhesiast, 42
Parsons, Talcott, 98
Pasolini, Pier Paolo, 100
past-present-future, 74
Patchen, Kenneth, 102
patient dumping, 152
patients, 30
  emotions, 32
  room, 31
  self-destructive, 38

unvaccinated, 38
Peeter, Benoit, 177
perception
  and the body, 59–60
  fabulation, 62
  game of fabulation, 61
  puzzle, 60–4
perceptual puzzles, 60–4
perpetual mourning, 150
pessimism, 91
Petty bureaucrats, 107
phantasms, 15
phantoms, 165, 166
Pharmakon, 81
Phenomenology of Perception, 59
Phenomenology of Spirit, 144, 173
phenomenology of study, 20
Phillips, Adam, 56
philosophers, 84, 196
  childhood, 163
  clock ticking, 173
  covid crisis, 163
  drain anxiety, 162
  "endless" nothingness, 164
  horrific pandemic, 168
  narrator, 172
  and psychoanalysts, 163
  psychoanalytic model, 166
  psycho-biographies, 162
Philosophical Investigations, 78
philosophical questions, 182
Philosophy of The Encounter, 189
Physicians, 34
  and the priest, 175–8
pieta, 92
Pinar, William F., 2, 3, 6, 21, 100, 173
plague, 180
  death, 174
  time, 174
The Plague (book), 161, 172–5
  authoritarianism, 180
  death-by-numbers, 180

metaphor, 180
plagues and pandemics, 180
Plato, 50
Poe, Edgar Allan, 48
Poetics (book), 50
poet-killers, 103
poetry-as-activism, 102
politicization, 5
pontificating, 78
Popper, Karl, 199
positivistic historiography, 55
postcolonial scholars, 184
poststructuralists, 42–3
power, 5
"precarious" stories, 24
presence as consciousness, 83
The Presence of the Dead, 181
The Primacy of Perception, 59
Prison Notebooks, 100
profanely-sacred sense, 72
professional philosophers, 177
prosopagnosia, 62
Protestant theology, 92
Proust, Marcel, 183
provincialism, 53
Psalm 23, 37
psyche, 141
psyche-somatic illnesses, 81
psychic wound, 204
psychoanalysis, 5, 6, 40, 57, 71, 112
psychological fantasies, 33
psychological reversal, 168
psychometrics, 98
psycho-pharmaceuticals, 141
psychoses, 141
psycho-somatic illness, 119, 120
puzzle, 60–4
puzzle-picture, 60–4
puzzles of perception, 133

Q

Questions of cosmology, 52
Questions of theology, 51
quest narrative, 41

R

Rabbi Joshua, 13
racism, 37
radical relativism, 75
Rahner, Karl, 68
raids, 91
Raids on the Unspeakable (book), 91
reaction-formation, 80
The Rebel, 10
rebellion, 17
Reck, Andrew, 50–53
Red Book, 16
refuge, 119
Reification, 96
religious cliches, 124
remembrance, 64
reorganization, 33
reparation, 167
reproducible teaching, 105
restitution narrative, 41
revelation, 116
revenants, 75, 83, 159
Rieux, Bernard, 172, 175, 176
rights of the unborn, 105
Rilke, Rainer Maria, 17
romantic science, 37–40, 43
Rome: The Book of Foundations, 199
Romero (film), 99
Ronell, Avital, 19, 143
Roosevelt, Teddy, 150
Ross, William, 194
The Rule of St. Benedict, 13–14
Russell, Bertrand, 98, 152, 179

228 | Index

Russia, 185

S

Sacks, Oliver, 37–40, 44, 56, 61, 133
The Sacred and the Profane, 72
sado-masochistic, 8
sage, 42
Sahara-like sky, 2
Saharan desert, 7
Said, Edward, 82, 98, 152
Salmon, Peter, 177
Salvio, Paula, 150
schism, 146
Schizophrenics, 15
Schnabel, Julian, 51
Schreber, Paul, 132
Science and Method, 191
second meditation, 17–20
self-actualization, 13
self-education, 182–3
self-organizing patterns, 190
Serres, Michel, 26, 76, 102, 106, 117, 121, 157, 202
  about plagues, 187
  absurdity, 188
  modern-day physics, 188
  the plague returns, 194
  theological disputations, 190
The Seven Storey Mountain, 14, 100
SF: Speculative Fabulation and String Figures (essay), 52
The Sheltering Sky, Saharan desert, 7, 8
shock therapy, 141
Shostakovich, Dmitri, 80
silence, 23
Silent Spring (book), 118
simultaneity, 47
Sintes, Catherine Helene, 164
Skeptics, 176

sleeping-sickness, 44–5
snow leopard, 66, 67
Socartes, 176
social constructions, 62
social psychology, 98
Socrates, 49–50, 77, 78, 115, 153
The Sopranos, 150
soul, 58
soul murder, 132
The South Central Review, 185
specters, 159
Specters of Marx, 75
speculation
  Aristotle, 49–51
  during covid, 63
  description, 48
  fabulation, 52, 62
  intellectual activity, 49, 63
  Latin verb, 48
  philosophy, 49
  psychological aspect, 57
  Socrates, 49–50
  Western philosophy, 63
speculative fabulation, 25, 47, 144
  chronicles, 53–4
  covid-19, 63
  pandemic, 62
  soul-work, 58
speculative reason, 142
speculum, in aenigmate (Latin phrase), 95
spirit, 142–4
The Spirit Catches You and You Fall Down, 41
spiritual content, 21
Stack, Liam, 13
states of horror, 54
statistics, 98
Stoic philosopher, 203
storytelling, 42–5, 52
stranger, 181–2
The Stranger, 169, 175
strife, contention, 195

string figures, 52
stripped-down rituals, 92
study and theory, 20–2
stultification
    chaplain, 32
    physician, 32
sublime, 9–10
Sweeney, Jon M., 12

T

taken-for-granted concept, 22
Tarkovsky, Andrey, 79
Tarrou, Jean, 172
teachers, 151, 195
techno-political stakes, 105
Ten Commandments, 150
Thales, 82
theological anthropology, 68
theological crisis, 3, 107
theology, 11
theoretical armature, 55
Theses on the Philosophy of History, 54
third meditation, 22–4
Three case histories: The "wolf man," the "rat man," and the psychotic doctor Schreber, 40
A Throw of the Dice Will Never Abolish Chance, 198
Thus Spoke Zarathustra, 192
Tikkun, 6
Tillich, Paul, 85
Todd, Olivier, 161, 182
tornadoes, 194
Torok, Maria, 165
total institution, 102
totalitarianism, 153
trace, 74–80
Tractatus, 52, 78
transcencendence, 72

transcendence, 95
transgenerational trauma, 166
transmarginal consciousness, 146
Trappist monks, 14, 91, 99, 102, 106
trauma, 55–6
traumatic situation, 171
Trifonas, Peter, 75
Trump, Donald John, 134
truth of absolutism, 178
truth-teller, 42
turbulence, 193
Turley, Hugh, 98
Turner, Jeff, 2
The Twilight of Idols, 202
Tyler, Ralph, 6
typologies, 42–5

U

unbearable stories, 47
    clinical chaplain, 113
    covid, 203–6
    curriculum studies, 24
    curriculum-writ-large, 23
    Didion, Joan, 126–31
    first-person witness, 112
    Jensen, Derrick, 132–7
    Marxism, 112
    Negative Dialectics, 111
    perspective, 113
    psychoanalysis, 112
    trauma literature, 114
    Williams, Terry Tempest, 117–26
unconscious, 30
universalisms, 81
universals, 81
unspeakable
    commons-of-covid, 89
    crisis, 90
unvaccination, 109
urgency, 76

Urrea, Luis Alberto, 9

V

vaccines, 62, 195
vanishing, 197–8
The Varieties of Religious Experience, 139
ventilation, 113
ventilators, 30, 203
verbatim, 31, 33, 34
Viallaneix, Paul, 168
via negativa, 108
violence, 66, 133
virus, 87
The Visible and the Invisible, 97
visual manifestation, 74
von Umwerth, Matthew, 17

W

Walden (2021), 107
Ward, Benedicta, 21
We alone are lost, 109, 110
Weatherhill, Rob, 21
Webb, David, 194
The Who and The What, 162
Why I am Not a Christian, 191
Williams, Terry Tempest, 2, 9, 25, 58, 60
    aporia, 118
    curriculum of unbearable stories, 114
    death on the horizon, 122–6
    denial, 122, 123
    family members, 117
    meaningless, 123
    mother, 124
    nonconceptualities, 121
    other's death, 124
    psychic Sibera, 126
    questioning politics, 118
    school children, 117
    slippery concepts, 121
    story, 119
    storytellers, 115
    women's cancers, 119
Will to Power, 99
Winnicott, D. W., 116, 141
without-hope-ness, 67
Wittgenstein, Antony, 22
Wittgenstein, Ludwig, 22, 60–4
work of mourning, 129
The worldliness of a cosmopolitan education: Passionate lives in public service, 6
The Wounded Storyteller, 25, 41
wreckage upon wreckage, 56
Wretched of the Earth, 184

Y

Year of Magical Thinking, 126

Z

Zarathustra, 92

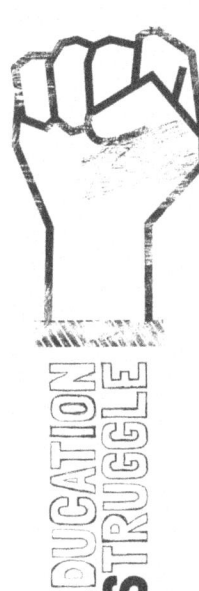

Narrative, Dialogue, and the Political Production of Meaning

Michael A. Peters
Peter McLaren
Series Editors

To submit a manuscript or proposal for editorial consideration, please contact:

Dr. Peter McLaren
Chapman University
College of Educational Studies
Reeves Hall 205
Orange, CA 92866

Dr. Michael A. Peters
University of Waikato
P.O. Box 3105
Faculty of Education
Hamilton 3240
New Zealand

WE ARE THE STORIES WE TELL. The book series Education and Struggle focuses on conflict as a discursive process where people struggle for legitimacy and the narrative process becomes a political struggle for meaning. But this series will also include the voices of authors and activists who are involved in conflicts over material necessities in their communities, schools, places of worship, and public squares as part of an ongoing search for dignity, self-determination, and autonomy. This series focuses on conflict and struggle within the realm of educational politics based around a series of interrelated themes: indigenous struggles; Western-Islamic conflicts; globalization and the clash of worldviews; neoliberalism as the war within; colonization and neocolonization; the coloniality of power and decolonial pedagogy; war and conflict; and the struggle for liberation. It publishes narrative accounts of specific struggles as well as theorizing "conflict narratives" and the political production of meaning in educational studies. During this time of global conflict and the crisis of capitalism, Education and Struggle promises to be on the cutting edge of social, cultural, educational, and political transformation.

Central to the series is the idea that language is a process of social, cultural, and class conflict. The aim is to focus on key semiotic, literary, and political concepts as a basis for a philosophy of language and culture where the underlying materialist philosophy of language and culture serves as the basis for the larger project that we might call dialogism (after Bakhtin's usage). As the late V. N. Volosinov suggests "Without signs there is no ideology," "Everything ideological possesses semiotic value," and "individual consciousness is a socio-ideological fact." It is a small step to claim, therefore, "consciousness itself can arise and become a viable fact only in the material embodiment of signs." This series is a vehicle for materialist semiotics in the narrative and dialogue of education and struggle.

To order other books in this series, please contact our Customer Service Department:

peterlang@presswarehouse.com (within the U.S.)
orders@peterlang.com (outside the U.S.)

Or browse online by series:

www.peterlang.com

www.ingramcontent.com/pod-product-compliance
Ingram Content Group UK Ltd.
Pitfield, Milton Keynes, MK11 3LW, UK
UKHW021327180426
11947UKWH00017B/1484